Practical Dementia Care

Practical Dementia Care

PETER V. RABINS, M.D., M.P.H.
CONSTANTINE G. LYKETSOS, M.D., M.H.S.
CYNTHIA D. STEELE, R.N., M.P.H.

School of Medicine
The Johns Hopkins University

New York   Oxford
OXFORD UNIVERSITY PRESS
1999

Oxford University Press

Oxford   New York
Athens   Auckland   Bangkok   Bogotá   Buenos Aires   Calcutta
Cape Town   Chennai   Dar es Salaam   Delhi   Florence   Hong Kong   Istanbul
Karachi   Kuala Lumpur   Madrid   Melbourne   Mexico City   Mumbai
Nairobi   Paris   São Paulo   Singapore   Taipei   Tokyo   Toronto   Warsaw

and associated companies in
Berlin   Ibadan

Copyright © 1999 by Peter V. Rabins, Constantine G. Lyketsos, Cynthia D. Steele

Published by Oxford University Press, Inc.,
198 Madison Avenue, New York, New York, 10016
http://www.oup-usa.org

Library of Congress Cataloging-in-Publication Data
Rabins, Peter V.
Practical dementia care / Peter V. Rabins, Constantine G. Lyketsos, Cynthia D. Steele.
p.   cm.   Includes bibliographical references.
ISBN 0-19-510625-3
1. Dementia—Patients—Care.
I. Lyketsos, Constantine G.
II. Steele, Cynthia, 1947–   .
III. Title.
[DNLM: 1. Dementia—therapy.
WM 220 R116p 1999]   RC521.R33   1999
616.8′3—dc21   DNLM/DLC   for Library of Congress   98-49715

The science of medicine is a rapidly changing field. As new research and clinical experience broaden our
knowledge, changes in treatment and drug therapy do occur. The author and the publisher of this work
have checked with sources believed to be reliable in their efforts to provide information that is accurate and
complete, and in accordance with the standards accepted at the time of publication. However, in light of the
possibility of human error or changes in the practice of medicine, neither the author, nor the publisher, nor
any other party who has been involved in the preparation or publication of this work warrants that the information contained herein is in every respect accurate or complete. Readers are encouraged to confirm the
information contained herein with other reliable sources, and are strongly advised to check the product information sheet provided by the pharmaceutical company for each drug they plan to administer.

3 4 5 6 7 8 9

Printed in the United States of America
on acid-free paper

To my family in appreciation of their care and support.
P. V. R.

To my father, my mother, and my wife,
the guiding lights of my life.
C. G. L.

To my husband for his steadfast support, and
to Jane Blaustein for her inspiration and enduring mentorship.
C. D. S.

Foreword

I am pleased to introduce readers to this book by my colleagues in the Department of Psychiatry at Johns Hopkins University School of Medicine. It furthers and enhances our long-standing commitment to the study and treatment of patients with dementing illnesses.

We are frequently asked about our dedication to patients with Alzheimer disease and other dementias—in particular why we see them as apt subjects for psychiatrists. The question prompts several responses from us that illuminate the responsibilities of contemporary psychiatrists.

Our initial response is to remind everyone that Aloys Alzheimer was a psychiatrist and, when he described the condition that bears his name, he was working in a psychiatric department and publishing his results in a psychiatric journal. Our contemporary commitment, though, might be considered outdated. After all Alzheimer's publications were some 90 years ago (the first in 1907). Surely psychiatry has changed its character and responsibilities since then—perhaps turning Alzheimer disease over to neurologists.

Our second response, however, is to acknowledge that psychiatry and neurology share an interest in dementia—psychiatrists because it is a mental disorder, neurologists because it is a brain disorder. Indeed, we celebrate that partnership here at Johns Hopkins by pointing to our local collaborative efforts that led to our recognizing how the neural degenerations in the Nucleus Basalis of Meynert and the Locus Ceruleus relate to the cognitive and affective symptoms of Alzheimer disease.

We do, though, remind everyone that long-term care for patients with dementia tends to be delivered by psychiatrists. Thus psychiatrists have been involved throughout this century in managing the clinical services of these patients in hospitals, nursing homes, and hospices. The knowledge that they have gained in these enterprises is illustrated in this book.

Although we work with other specialists such as geriatricians and neurologists, we do not take a back seat to them in our practice, teaching, or research. We hold that our commitments to these patients have helped advance their treatment. In particular, we identified how the settings where these patients receive care are best viewed as psychiatric centers deserving—indeed requiring—the services, resources, and milieu management that protect patients from emotional and behavioral unrest. This book demonstrates just how diagnostic formulations and treatment planning are managed in many different settings with benefit to patients.

We hold that this commitment to the study and care of demented patients—outlined so effectively in this book—helped us demonstrate new implications for psychiatry as a specialty of medicine. The twentieth century has seen medicine and surgery turn to biology for their justifications—with biology understood as the study of life. This idea did more than just bring new treatments to light, it brought forth the fundamental concept that physical illnesses are best construed as "life under altered circumstances" rather than dehumanizing distinctions or harbingers of mortality. Just so do we appreciate psychiatric conditions such as dementia, as human life under altered circumstances—here of cerebral disruptions—and the patients who live under these circumstances as humans in need of support and care.

This concept spurns the view that these patients are defined by their diagnosis or that they should be removed to places where exertions in their service can be minimized. It underscores that these patients are fundamentally the same as any medically ill people—humans living under altered circumstances that the rest of us can make better or worse depending upon our understanding.

Indeed, service to these patients led us to challenge the over-emphasis in contemporary medical ethics on human autonomy versus human interdependence—a rhetorical emphasis that regularly disputes the utility of the effort we wish to expend on these patients and occasionally has encouraged their neglect. From working with patients we have learned to stress that the recognition of human interdependence is the starting point for coherent ethics just as it is for a coherent psychiatry to advocate for the mentally ill.

Psychiatrists see interdependence as the fundamental human social characteristic and note its role in family life, professional pursuits, and institutions—interdependence represented by the network of responsibilities within which all people live and from which their autonomy emerges. Patients with Alzheimer dementia, are increasingly and inexorably dependent on others over time but respond, with enhanced capabilities and reduced emotional distress, to the attention and treatment described in these pages. They demonstrate how autonomy can be a result of care, rather than a distinct attribute of patients that defines who is entitled to care and who is not.

As psychiatrists envision dementing patients as humans specially burdened by altered circumstances, they appreciate a duty to learn about those circumstances and to stress how efforts on behalf of these patients can ease their burdens and will eventually bring knowledge to cure them. Here research, practice, and ethics combine—all emphasizing the primacy of human interdependence in our endeavors. This book demonstrates how it is done.

Paul R. McHugh, M.D.
Henry Phipps Professor and Director
Department of Psychiatry and Behavioral Sciences
The Johns Hopkins University

Acknowledgments

We wish to thank Paul McHugh, M.D., Jason Brandt, Ph.D., Susan Kopunek, B.S.N., Martin Steinberg, M.D., Andrew Warren, M.D., Alva Baker, M.D., Carol Kershner, M.S.W., Carmel Rogues, M.S.W., Elizabeth Galik, R.N., the clinical team of the Johns Hopkins Neuropsychiatry and Memory Group, and the staff at Copper Ridge for their contributions over the years to the development of Practical Dementia Care. We also wish to thank Karen Rabins for carefully editing the manuscript, and Betty Burgeois for her work in typing the manuscript.

Contents

Practical Dementia Care

Introduction

Dementia care has entered a new era. Advances in epidemiology, neuroscience, and our understanding of brain–behavior relationships have all contributed to this. The search for the causes of dementia intensified in the 1990s, and new treatments are being studied daily. The focus is slowly expanding to add prevention, early diagnosis, and rational treatment over the course of the illness.

The public health importance and societal costs associated with dementia make effective treatment a primary concern for everyone: the patient, the family, the medical community, and society at large. The number and background of persons involved in the care of dementia patients are expanding. Physicians, nurses, psychologists, social workers, rehabilitation therapists, activity specialists, long-term care specialists, and, as always, family caregivers are now included. A good understanding of dementia coupled with a rational, systematic approach to the care of the dementia patient is essential for clinicians. A "can-do" attitude and an approach that views persons with dementia as people who can be helped, whose life can be made better and whose family can be effectively supported are crucial to the success of this enterprise. This rehabilitation model stresses accurate diagnosis and assessment; the identification of patient, caregiver, and environmental characteristics that are amenable to treatment; and an acknowledgment that disease imposes some limits that cannot be overcome.

This book is intended to provide a common language, attitude, and treatment approach for clinicians involved in dementia care. It defines principles and interweaves them with systematic and practical ways of caring for dementia patients throughout the stages and complexities of the disorder.

This book is meant to be used in day-to-day practice by all groups of professionals involved in the evaluation and treatment of people who suffer from one of the many disorders that cause dementia. It takes a broad, holistic approach to dementia and should be useful to professionals treating patients in settings varying from the community to the hospital. It may be of particular interest to professionals caring for people with dementia who reside in long-term care facilities such as retirement communities, assisted living facilities, and nursing homes. We hope that the book is also useful to policymakers, health administrators, and others who want to understand the skills involved in providing care for people with dementia.

Caring for people with dementia is very challenging. One must consider the disorder and the ill person from several different viewpoints. Paul McHugh and Phillip Slavney have suggested that four perspectives guide the clinician's approach. First, all will agree that the cardinal disturbance of dementia, the cognitive disorder, results from an impairment of brain function. This must be the starting point and is called the *disease perspective*. Second, the disease afflicts a person who has attributes that she or he has carried throughout life—personality traits, innate cognitive abilities, likes and dislikes, skills and interests. These are universal characteristics of human beings and are best considered as graded dimensions because people differ in amount or extent of the characteristic. *Dimensional characteristics* of people with dementia are important to consider since they shape the person's symptoms, reactions, and behaviors. In addition, these essential characteristics of a person are sometimes changed by the disease. For example, a person who has been suspicious and irritable might become pleasant and trusting. Prompting the family to describe a patient's characteristics before the development of his or her illness can help the clinician appreciate how the patient is responding to the illness and also how the family is reacting to its manifestations.

A very different viewpoint shapes the third perspective on dementia care. At the level of behavior, we become less interested in the cause of a problem and focus more on helping the person adapt more comfortably to the problems imposed by the disease. Problems in behavior are common in persons with dementia and will be extensively discussed in Chapters 8 and 9. The ability to take a *behavioral approach* is one of the most important requirements in a professional providing care for individuals with dementia. It requires a set of skills that can be learned and taught.

The fourth perspective, the *life story approach,* requires the professional caregiver to understand the uniqueness of each individual who is suffering from dementia and to appreciate the many meanings that these illnesses carry with them. The ability to understand the fear and sense of loss experienced by many patients with dementia and by their loved ones complements the other three viewpoints (or perspectives) and is as necessary as they are for providing good care.

The challenge is clear. Professionals who dedicate themselves to caring for individuals with dementia must be willing to think at multiple levels. The artificial boundaries imposed by profession (nurse, doctor, social worker, activity therapist) and model of care (medical model, social model, holistic model) break down in the face of complex diseases like the dementias. A major challenge faced by students, practitioners, policymakers, and planners is that each approach and each profession makes unique contributions to the care of people with dementia. The skillful provider is the person who can move from one mode of thinking to another, depending on the circumstances.

The difficulties and challenges of caring for individuals with dementia should not be underestimated or exaggerated. The rewards of providing care are many. They are based on the improved quality of life that good professional care brings to the ill, their family members, their loved ones, and to society as a whole. This book is built upon the belief that the best care is provided by individuals who are well trained, who have developed a variety of techniques, who treat each patient as an individual, and who are able to identify, within themselves, the rewards and frustrations of caring for people with chronic and usually progressive debilitating diseases.

Definitions and Overview of the Book

Dementia is a clinical syndrome caused by a wide range of diseases that affect the brain. Its core feature is a decline in cognition. Dementia has many presentations as well as causes. It can be stable or progressive. It can afflict the young or the old. It is associated with a wide range of mental and behavioral disturbances, many of which are reminiscent of other psychiatric disorders. Dementia involves functional impairments that derive from the impairments in cognition but can also result from behavioral disturbances. Dementia renders individuals more vulnerable to the effects of coexisting medical conditions and medications. Finally, dementia occurs in a family context and affects the lives of many others. Caring for the dementia patient is a complex endeavor. It requires several skills and the involvement of the patient, family, care providers, and health professionals.

This first chapter introduces definitions that professionals caring for patients with dementia need to keep in mind. We discuss the magnitude, burdens, and costs of dementia and then the complexities of dementia care. Finally, the book's organization is described.

DEFINITIONS

Dementia

The word *dementia* derives from the Latin *de mens* and means "from the mind." Its mention in the Bible and in early Egyptian, Greek, and Roman writings suggests that it has affected humankind since the dawn of time. To many, the word *dementia* implies craziness, irrationality, and hopelessness. None of these is an accurate description of the syndrome. Many terms have been proposed to replace the word *dementia,* but all have acquired the same undesirable connotations. This suggests that it is not the word that is frightening but the disorder it describes. Dementia is best defined as a *syndrome,* a pattern of clinical symptoms and signs that meets the criteria presented in Table 1.1. The first element of the definition is a decline, or deterioration, in the cognitive or thinking capacities. This decline from a previous level of ability distinguishes dementia from disorders of cognition that have been present since birth—for example, mental retardation and learning disabilities.

The second element of the definition requires that more than one area of cognition be impaired. Memory is affected by almost every disease that causes dementia; the other cognitive impairments in judgment, perception, language, abstraction, persistence, and calculation depend on the specific disease and the stage of the illness. This criterion distinguishes dementia from disorders in which only a single cognitive ability is impaired, such as aphasia, in which language disorder is present, and the amnestic syndrome, in which only memory is impaired.

Even though dementia requires multiple impairments, not all cognitive functions are necessarily affected. In addition, the functions that are impaired often vary in the degree to which they are involved. Thus, there is variation from patient to patient in the type and severity of cognitive processes that are impaired. The identification of retained capacities is an important component of treatment planning that can help the ill person remain as functional as possible.

Based on the pattern of cognitive impairment (phenomenology), two types of dementia syndromes are recognized, the cortical type and the subcortical type. In the cortical type the brain pathology predominantly affects cognitive functions that are located in the outside layers of the brain, the cortex, such as memory, language, gnosis, and praxis. Loss of memory capacity is called *amnesia*; language impairment is referred to as *aphasia*; impairment in the ability to do learned motor tasks is called *apraxia*; and impairment in pattern recognition is called *agnosia*. Thus, the cortical dementias are characterized by amnesia, aphasia, apraxia, and agnosia (the four A's). Alzheimer disease is the best example. In

Table 1.1. Definition of Dementia

1. Decline of cognitive capacity (memory, language, judgment, etc.)

2. Multiple areas of cognition impaired (global)

3. Normal level of consciousness (absence of delirium)

subcortical dementia the pathology involves primarily deeper brain structure. Patients lose the ability to coordinate cognition and have difficulties with memory (forgetfulness), slowed thinking and moving, trouble with decisionmaking, and reduced complexity of thought (dysmnesia, delay, dysexecutive, and depletion—the four D's). Of note, cortical and subcortical disturbances can coexist, in which case patients are said to have "mixed" dementia.

Table 1.2 summarizes the distinction between cortical and subcortical dementia. Patients with cortical dementia lose cognitive capacities, the ability to "do." In contrast, patients with subcortical dementia lose the ability to coordinate cognition but often retain the ability to "do" it. A parallel from motor disturbances is apt: Patients with a stroke in the motor area lose the ability to "do" movement (cortical) while patients with Parkinson disease can "do" movement but are unable to coordinate it properly, so their movements are delayed, slowed, imprecise, or lack in dexterity (subcortical).

The third element of the definition of dementia is that alertness and awakeness are not impaired. This criterion is sometimes stated as having "a normal level of consciousness" and distinguishes dementia from delirium. *Delirium* is a condition in which the patient is drowsy, inattentive, or unable to sustain concentration, and in which multiple impairments in thinking are present. Delirium usually begins suddenly and is often associated with disordered sleep, visual hallucinations, and behavior change.

Table 1.2. Cortical Versus Subcortical Dementia

	Cortical	Subcortical
Key feature	Loss of core ability (capacity) to "do" cognition	Loss of ability to coordinate cognition
Mnemonic	The four *A*'s	The four *D*'s
Features	Amnesia Apraxia Agnosia Aphasia	Dysmnesia Dysexecutive Delay Depletion
Typical symptoms	Can't recall or recognize	Benefits from cues to remember
	Repeats questions	Thinking/movement are slowed
	Can't do things	Trouble planning and executing
	Doesn't "know" things	Less flexible
	Trouble with language	Less initiative

Delirium is most commonly caused by a metabolic abnormality (such as abnormal electrolytes), an infectious process, medication toxicity or a combination of causes. Dementia and delirium often occur together because dementia is a risk factor for developing delirium. Since delirium is often reversible, its recognition should lead to an intensive search for a cause.

It can be difficult to distinguish between delirium and dementia when memory or language is so severely impaired that the patient is unable to sustain a conversation, or when perceptual dysfunction is so marked that the patient seems not to "pay attention" to other people or to the environment. If they are fully alert, they do not meet the "altered level of consciousness" criteria of delirium.

The frequent co-occurrence of delirium and dementia was illustrated by a large Finnish study in which 2,000 individuals were examined on admission to a general hospital. Fifteen percent of the patients over age 55 suffered from delirium. Twenty-five percent of this group were later found to be suffering from an underlying dementia, twice the rate of dementia in nondelirious admissions. Among those who developed delirium while hospitalized, 22% suffered from dementia.

Dementia is caused by a disease of the brain. By disease we mean a process that causes something to be broken in the structure or function of the brain. This might be from a direct mechanical injury, such as trauma, from degeneration or death of brain cells, or from a factor that temporarily disrupts brain cell function such as dementia caused by abnormal levels of thyroid hormones. These pathologic changes can have one or several causes. Ultimately, every dementia syndrome will be associated with a specific pathologic change due to a specific disease. The location and extent of the damage to the brain will explain the symptom profile (the syndrome) in many cases. Table 1.3 lists the most common diseases that cause dementia.

Noncognitive Symptoms

Behavioral and psychiatric disturbances refer to a wide range of disorders in mental life and behavior which afflict some patients with dementia. These are defined descriptively, sometimes as individual symptoms and at other times as syndromes. The most common such disturbances are listed on Table 1.4 (for definitions see the Glossary). In this book we shall use the terms *behavioral disturbances* and *noncognitive symptoms* interchangeably to mean both mental and behavioral disorders. In some instances, the disease causing the dementia also injures brain areas which are important to the regulation of mood and behavior. In other cases, the behavioral disturbances are a consequence of the cognitive disorder itself. Additionally, these behavioral disturbances might be the

Table 1.3. Dementia-Causing Diseases

Degenerative Brain Diseases
Alzheimer disease
Parkinson disease
Pick disease
Frontotemporal degeneration
Huntington disease
Progressive supranuclear palsy
Spinocerebellar degenerations
Multiple sclerosis

Cerebrovascular Diseases
Multiple infarct disease
Binswanger disease
Subcortical leukoareosis
Thalamic infarct

Cerebral Vasculitides
Lupus erythematosus
Temporal arteritis
Giant cell arteritis

Infectious Diseases
Syphilis (general paresis of the insane)
Tuberculosis
HIV disease (AIDS dementia complex)
Prion diseases (Creutzfeld-Jakob disease)
Fungal encephalitides
Viral encephalitides

Psychiatric Disorders
Major depressive disorder
Schizophrenia

Traumatic Brain Injuries
Closed head injury
Open head injury
Subdural hematoma

Vitamin Deficiencies
Vitamin B_{12} deficiency (subacute combined sclerosis, pernicious anemia)
Vitamin B_6 deficiency (pellagra)
Vitamin B_1 (Thiamine) deficiency

Endocrine Diseases
Hyperthyroidism
Hypothyroidism
Growth hormone deficiency
Hyperparathyroidism
Cushing disease (hyperadrenalism)
Conn disease (hypoadrenalism)

Cerebral Tumors
Intrinsic brain tumor
Metastatic cancer

Toxin Exposure
Alcohol
Heavy metals (lead, arsenic, mercury)
Volatile hydrocarbons
Medications

Other
Normal pressure (communicating) hydrocephalus

consequence of preexisting psychiatric disorders or may be due to co-morbid medical problems or medications which dementia patients are receiving (for more detail see Chapters 8 and 9).

The importance of mental and behavioral disturbances in dementia is underscored by their high prevalence and high morbidity. Some 25%–40% of patients with mild dementia and as many as 75%–80% of patients with severe dementia, particularly those who are institutionalized or in nursing homes, suffer from them. In addition, these disturbances contribute to the disability experienced by dementia patients. For example, problems as diverse as depression, hallucinations, and irritability might prevent a person from participating in daycare programs even if they have the cognitive and physical capacities to do so. Furthermore, behavioral disturbances contribute to the burnout of caregivers. This is one of the main reasons dementia patients are placed in long-term care facilities.

Table 1.4. Noncognitive Disturbances
in Dementia

Delirium

Mood Disturbances
  Depression
  Anxiety
  Irritability
  Mania

Suspiciousness, Paranoia, and Delusions

Hallucinations and Illusions

Problem Behaviors
  Catastrophic reactions
  Rummaging and hoarding
  Aggression/agitation
  Wandering and pacing
  Yelling, calling out, and screaming
  Social withdrawal and apathy
  Catastrophic reactions
  Uncooperativeness and resistance to care

Disturbance of Basic Drives
  Sexual disorders
  Sleep disorders
  Disorders of eating, weight, or appetite

Impairment and Disability

The losses of function associated with dementia range from very mild to
very severe. Relatively mild impairments include the inability to carry-
out instrumental activities of daily living (IADLs) such as working,
maintaining a living space, shopping, cleaning house, handling money,
using the telephone, getting from place to place, driving, and so forth.
Almost all patients with dementia have impairments in some of these
instrumental activities and most are dependent on others for all of these
activities. As the dementia progresses (or in more severe cases), patients
lose the ability to carry out more basic activities of daily living (ADLs),
such as dressing, bathing, personal care, toileting, navigating in their
home, and eating. An additional source of disability for some patients
is losing the ability to self-regulate. This results in doing things that are
inappropriate, socially objectionable, or dangerous, such as, wandering and getting lost, hitting others who try to help them with daily
activities, sitting in one place all day, becoming deconditioned (losing
stamina, muscle tone and mass, and so on), and being at high risk
for falling. Table 1.5 provides one approach to staging functional im-

pairment, the FAST system of Reisberg and collaborators. This was developed for Alzheimer disease (AD) but is applicable to other dementias as well.

Comorbidity.

Dementia patients are very vulnerable to illness and many suffer from other medical and psychiatric disorders. The explanation for this is not clear but may have to do with the fact that dementia results in widespread disease of the brain. Another factor is the association between old age and chronic illnesses such as arthritis and diabetes, but the main reason is probably that brain dysfunction lowers the threshold for developing symptoms. For example, an elderly patient without dementia is better able to handle the flu than an elderly person with dementia. Dementia also makes patients more likely to develop side effects from medications.

The presence of comorbid medical illness or the use of medications in dementia patients often results in a worsening of cognitive symptoms, the development of delirium, the onset of behavioral symptoms, or further decline. The provision of good medical, surgical, dental, gynecologic, and psychiatric care to dementia patients is critical for minimizing the effects of comorbidity.

Caregivers.

Given the disabilities associated with dementia, all patients with dementia need some assistance. The degree of caregiver involvement is usually proportional to the level of impairment and disability that the patient has. The majority of dementia caregivers are family members, usually women, who are spouses, adult children, or siblings. Chapter 7 discusses their needs and the needs of professional caregivers.

THE SCOPE OF THE PROBLEM

Epidemiologists study the occurrence of a disorder in the population. They seek to discover the causes of disease by determining how the condition is distributed in the population; they try to identify protective and risk factors; and they study treatment and prevention strategies.

Prevalence refers to the number of cases of a condition in a population. Before age 65, the prevalence of dementia is low, on the order of five to 10 per 1,000 people (0.5%–1%). In this younger age group, dementia is most commonly caused by head injuries. Brain diseases such as multiple sclerosis, Alzheimer disease, toxic disorders, infections such as encephalitis can also cause dementia in the young and others.

Table 1.5. FAST STAGES

FAST Stage	Characteristics	Clinical Diagnosis
1	No objective or subjective functional decrement	Normal adult
2	Subjective deficit in recalling names or other word finding and/or subjective deficit in recalling location of objects and/or subjectively decreased ability to recall appointments. No objectively manifest functional deficits	Normal-aged adult
3	*Deficits noted in demanding occupational and social settings* (e.g., the individual may begin to forget important appointments for the first time; work productivity may decline); problems may be noted in traveling to unfamiliar locations (e.g., may get lost traveling by automobile and/or public transportation to a "new" location or spot)	Compatible with incipient AD
4	*Deficits in performance of complex tasks of daily life* (e.g., paying bills and/or balancing checkbook; decreased capacity in planning and/or preparing an elaborate meal; decreased capacity in marketing, such as in the correct purchase of grocery items)	Mild AD
5	*Deficient performance in choosing proper attire, and assistance is required for independent community functioning*—the spouse or other caregiver frequently must help the individual choose the appropriate clothing for the occasion and/or season (e.g., the individual will wear incongruous clothing); over the course of this stage some patients may also begin to forget to bathe regularly (unless reminded) and automobile driving ability becomes compromised (e.g., carelessness in driving in automobile and violations of driving rules)	Moderate AD
6a	*Requires actual physical assistance in putting on clothing properly*—the caregiver must provide increasing assistance with the actual mechanics of helping the individual clothe himself properly (e.g., putting on clothing in the proper sequence, tying shoelaces, putting shoes on proper feet, buttoning and/or zipping clothing, putting on blouse, shirt, pants, skirt, etc., correctly)	Moderately severe AD
6b	*Requires assistance bathing properly*—the patient's ability to adjust bathwater temperature diminishes; the patient may have difficulty entering and leaving the bath; there may be problems with washing properly and completely drying oneself	Moderately severe AD
6c	*Requires assistance with mechanics of toileting*—patients at this stage may forget to flush the toilet and	Moderately severe AD

may begin to wipe themselves improperly or less fastidiously when toileting

6d	*Urinary incontinence*—this occurs in the absence of infection or other genitourinary tract pathology; the patient has episodes of urinary incontinence. Frequency of toileting may mitigate the occurrence of incontinence somewhat	Moderately severe AD
6e	*Fecal incontinence*—in the absence of gastrointestinal pathology, the patient has episodes of fecal incontinence. Frequency of toileting may mitigate the occurrence of incontinence somewhat	Moderately severe AD
7a	*Speech limited to about six words in the course of an average day*—during the course of an average day the patient's speech is restricted to single words (e.g., "Yes," "No," "Please") or short phrases (e.g., "Please don't hurt me"; "Get away"; "Get out of here"; "I like you")	Severe AD
7b	*Intelligible vocabulary limited to generally a single word in the course of an average day*—as the illness progresses the ability to utter even short phrases on a regular basis is lost so that the spoken vocabulary becomes limited to generally one or two single words as an indicator for all things and needs (e.g., "Yes," "No," "O.K." for all verbalization-provoking phenomena)	Severe AD
7c	*Ambulatory ability lost*—patients gradually lose the ability to ambulate independently; in the early part of this substage they may require actual support (e.g., being physically supported by a caregiver) and physical assistance to walk, but as the substage progresses, the ability to ambulate even with assistance is lost; the onset is somewhat varied with some patients simply taking progressively smaller and slower steps—other patients begin to tilt forward, backward or laterally when ambulating; twisted gaits have also been noted as antecedents of ambulatory loss	Severe AD
7d	*Ability to sit up lost*—the patients lose the ability to sit up without assistance(e.g., they need some form of physical brace—an armrest, a belt, or other brace or other special devices to keep them from sliding down in the chair)	Severe AD
7e	*Ability to smile lost*—patients are no longer observed to smile, although they do manifest other facial movements and sometimes grimace	Severe AD
7f	*Ability to hold head up lost*—patients can no longer hold up their head unless the head is supported	Severe AD

Adapted from Reisberg, B. (1986). *Geriatrics,* 41:30-46

Over age 65, the prevalence of dementia increases dramatically (Figure 1.1). Among people 65 years of age and older, 50–80 per 1,000 (5%–8%) suffer from dementia. This number increases to 180–200 per 1,000 (18%–20%) for those 75 and older and to 350–400 per 1,000 (35%–40%) for individuals 85 years of age and older. Over age 65, Alzheimer disease is the cause of 60%–70% of dementia.

The prevalence of dementia depends on the age distribution of the population. Currently, in the United States, there are 3 to 4 million people with dementia, most of whom are elderly. This number will increase dramatically over the next few decades because the number of people living to old age is increasing. As a result, the number of people with dementia is expected to double by the year 2020 unless a prevention or cure is developed for at least one of the common causes. The most rapidly growing age group is that of individuals 85 years old or older, the "very old" group in which Alzheimer disease is most prevalent. This is the primary reason that the number of people with dementia will increase so dramatically.

The incidence rate of dementia also increases with age. Incidence is defined as the number of new cases of a disorder occurring in a given period of time. At age 65, an individual who does not have dementia, has a 2.5 per 1,000 (0.25%) chance of developing dementia during the next year. This rate approximately doubles every 5 years (Figure 1.2) so that by age 70, an individual who does not have dementia has a 5 per 1,000 (0.5%) chance of developing dementia in the next year. By age 85, the annual incidence rate is 4%. Thus, the longer one lives, the greater the chance one has of developing dementia. Furthermore, as average life expectancy increases, the risk of developing dementia increases since living longer means living to an age at which the incidence rate is higher.

Data on incidence are available only up to age 90. We do not know yet what happens to people who live into their 90's and 100's. Several possibilities can be imagined. In one, the trend will continue, with the incidence doubling every 5 years. If this in fact is true, and the incidence continues to rise through the life span, then almost every individual will develop dementia by age 112. An alternative possibility is that the incidence rate of dementia peaks at age 90 or 95 and then stabilizes or begins to decline. Recent data from the Cache County Memory Study in Utah suggest that the prevalence of dementia may stabilize after age 85, but other studies will need to confirm this.

Another way of looking at the scope of dementia is to examine its cost to society. Direct costs, estimated at 80 billion dollars per year in the U.S., relate to the direct provision of care to people with dementia.

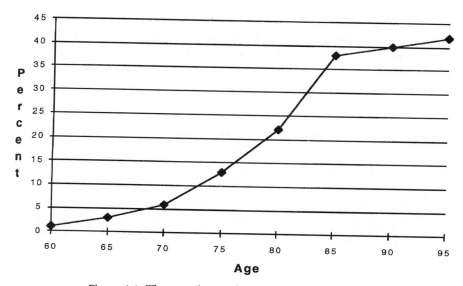

Figure 1.1. The prevalence of dementia at different ages.

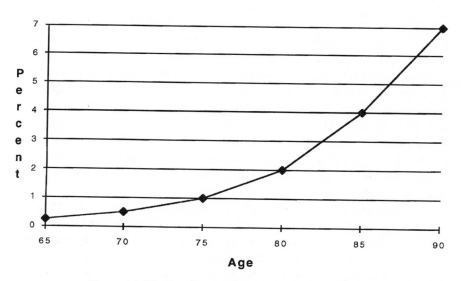

Figure 1.2. The incidence of dementia at different ages.

Indirect costs, which result from non-medical expenses, probably represent an additional 20–30 billion dollars per year. They include the health care costs of caregivers, the years of productive life lost by the patient, and the loss of productivity of caregivers, due to missing work or retiring early, for example.

THE COMPLEXITIES OF DEMENTIA CARE

Professionals who care for patients with dementia need to be aware of the diverse presentations of dementia, the variety of treatments that are available, and the importance of social, environmental, medical, and psychological issues. Dementia care can be provided at a variety of geographic locations but the care needs to be coordinated among these sites.

Patients with progressive dementia require day-to-day structure, protection from victimization, and good medical care. As the dementia progresses, patients lose their capacity for independent decisionmaking; others must make decisions for them. They will lose the ability to drive and live alone. Each of these losses adds a layer of complexity.

Dementia care involves providing support to family members and other care-providers, and this includes helping them understand the patient's symptoms and condition, helping them care for the patient, and helping them gain access to resources. Additionally, family care-providers require considerable emotional support because day-to-day caregiving is taxing and emotionally devastating.

Families, particularly children, of dementia patients also have another major concern. They have to live with the question, "Is this likely to happen to me?" This arises from the recognition that they will grow old and may suffer a similar dementing illness, and from evolving knowledge reported in the mass media that certain dementias are heritable. Having a parent or other relative with dementia clearly affects a child's risk of getting it, perhaps at a younger age than expected in the general population.

Professional care-providers are confronted with caring for patients with a complex, multifaceted, relentless disease, often terminal in nature. Cognitive, behavioral, and functional impairments all occur and incapacitate patients and families. They need to understand the various diseases that cause dementia, be prepared to detect it early, keep up with new scientific information about dementia, and maintain stamina and hope in the face of the cruelty of the disease. These needs make the task of dementia care a challenging one for the professional.

HOW TO USE THIS BOOK

The discussion above illustrates how challenging dementia care can be. We believe that it is possible to go about it systematically, in a way that maximizes benefits to patients and families and that sustains the interest and warmth of the professional care-provider, thus preventing burnout. This book is intended to be a practical source and reference for the professional providing day-to-day care to patients. It is not written as a comprehensive reference work. We have forgone systematic referencing in order to make the book more user-friendly. We have included many tables and figures as well as practical aids to management, such as checklists, for use in day-to-day practice with dementia patients.

The organization of this book is as follows. The overview of dementia in this chapter is complemented by the glossary at the end of the book. Chapter 2 describes the process of evaluating and formulating a case of suspected dementia. Chapters 3 and 4 cover the basic facts about the most common dementia-causing diseases. Many of these facts will change over time as new knowledge is gained about dementia and the different diseases which cause it. However, some basic issues such as definitions and complexities of care are unlikely to change. The same is true of the practical approaches to evaluation and treatment presented throughout the book.

Chapter 5 provides a systematic overview of dementia care, organized to include principles, goals, and the development of treatment plans. The next two chapters (6 and 7) discuss in detail the supportive care that must be provided to patients and to caregivers. Chapters 8 and 9 focus on problem solving and discuss a long list of clinical problems frequently encountered in dementia care. For each of these, the chapters provide a definition of the problem and specific approaches to addressing it. Chapter 8 deals with problems arising from behavioral or psychiatric disturbances associated with dementia and Chapter 9 deals with problems that arise directly out of impairments in functioning (such as bathing, dressing, and driving) or problems with eating, sleeping, and sexuality. Chapter 10 provides an overview of currently available medications and other biologic strategies that might be used with dementia patients. Chapter 11 discusses care for patients in the late stages of dementia. Chapter 12 offers practical approaches to legal and ethical issues that arise in dementia care. Chapter 13 presents a genetics primer and an approach to providing genetic counseling for patients with dementia and their family members.

Professionals who read this book are strongly encouraged to augment their day-to-day practice with ongoing education about dementia care such as a subscription to professional newsletters that relate to dementia and participation in groups that advocate better care of and research into dementia. These include the Alzheimer Association, the Parkinsons Disease Society of America, and the Brain Injury Association.

The Evaluation and Formulation of Dementia

*T*his chapter discusses the evaluation of a patient with memory complaints or suspected dementia. The first part of the chapter discusses the following questions: (1) When should a comprehensive dementia evaluation be performed? (2) What is the purpose of such an evaluation? (3) Who is involved in performing such an evaluation? (4) What is the process of this evaluation?

The second part of the chapter discusses how to perform an assessment of a person with suspected dementia. Chapter 5 discusses how to use the information from the assessment in the differential diagnosis and workup of dementia.

BACKGROUND

When Should a "Comprehensive" Dementia Evaluation Be Performed?

In most cases the recognition that an evaluation is needed does not come from the patient. Typically, a family member, such as a spouse or a child, notices forgetfulness, communication difficulty, problems functioning, or a personality change and persuades the patient to be evaluated. Primary care physicians, neurologists or psychiatrists, and specialists in dementia are often the first professionals to see patients.

This reliance on family members and patients to recognize dementia often leads to delays in diagnosis. Of the patients seen for an initial evaluation at the Johns Hopkins Comprehensive Alzheimer Program, only 15%–20% are in the early stages of the disease and one-third are in the late stages of dementia. More often than not, evaluations are sought when crises occur such as dangerous behavior, forgetting to pay bills, having a car accident, withdrawing from social activities, or stopping activities such as cooking.

There are several benefits of early diagnosis. First, the functional decline of dementia and its consequences can be better managed if anticipated and addressed early. For example, financial catastrophes and injuries from car accidents or falls can be prevented by the knowledge that the patient is impaired. Second, early identification helps the family and patient understand changes in behavior and judgment that are often early symptoms. Behavioral disorders such as depression, delusions, and aggression are more likely to respond to treatment if caught early and treated appropriately. Third, early diagnosis allows patients and families more time for long-range planning to manage the consequences of dementia. This includes the ability to do estate planning, appoint a power of attorney (Chapter 12), and so forth. Fourth, early diagnosis may improve the response to treatments for the cognitive symptoms or delay progression in some diseases.

Despite this, we do not believe widespread screening of asymptomatic individuals can be justified at present. In the future, when more effective therapies are available and treatments that are preventative are developed, screening evaluations of at-risk individuals will be warranted.

In order to improve recognition and early diagnosis of dementia we recommend that an evaluation be considered for elderly persons and other persons with neurologic disease or head injury who develop any of the signs or symptoms listed in Table 2.1.

Of the problems listed on the table, memory impairment and impaired functioning are most likely to be ascribed to normal aging and be explained away or ignored. Since there are slight declines in cognition and functioning associated with aging, awareness of usual aging changes is necessary. For example, difficulty remembering names or coming up with the right word without any of the other symptoms in Table 2.1 is unlikely to be due to dementia. One piece of information that is especially useful in the primary care setting is a standardized cognitive assessment done during routine medical checkups. Tools such as the Mini-Mental State Examination (MMSE) are available and can be administered annually or biannually in less than 10 minutes by a physician or other health professional. A decline of more than three points on the MMSE from a stable baseline should trigger an evaluation.

What Are the Purposes of a Dementia Evaluation?

The primary purpose of the dementia evaluation is to determine whether dementia is present or absent. Dementia is a clinical diagnosis

Table 2.1. Signs and Symptoms Which Should Trigger Consideration of a Dementia Evaluation

1. Cognitive Changes
New forgetfulness, more trouble understanding spoken and written communication, difficulty finding words, not knowing things the person should know (such as the president or where they are), disorientation

2. Psychiatric Symptoms
Withdrawal or apathy, depression, suspiciousness, anxiety, insomnia, fearfulness, paranoia, abnormal beliefs, hallucinations

3. Personality Changes
Inappropriate friendliness, blunting and disinterest, social withdrawal, excessive flirtatiousness, easy frustration, explosive spells

4. Problem Behaviors
Wandering, agitation, noisiness, restlessness, being out of bed at night

5. Changes in Day-to-Day Functioning
Difficulty driving, getting lost, forgetting recipes in cooking, neglecting selfcare, neglecting household chores, difficulty handling money, making mistakes at work, trouble with shopping

which depends on the demonstration of a global decline in cognitive capacity in clear consciousness. The evaluation may demonstrate that dementia is not present and that the complaints or concerns which initiated the evaluation can be attributed to some other cause such as usual aging, depression, a previously unrecognized neurologic or medical condition such as Parkinson disease, hypothyroidism, alcohol abuse, or medication side effects.

If dementia is identified, the next step is to ascertain the cause of the dementia syndrome. This is a necessary step in determining both the most appropriate treatment and the likely prognosis—another purpose of the assessment is the identification of remaining abilities and disabilities that result from the dementia. This too has an important influence on the treatment plan. Finally, the evaluation lays the groundwork for developing a plan of care. It determines the kinds of information, guidance, and emotional support the patient and family require to deal with a chronic illness.

Who Is Involved in Performing a Dementia Evaluation?

Most dementia assessments can be accomplished in the community in primary care settings. Specialists are best used when the diagnosis is in question, the case is atypical, the symptoms are complex or initial management strategies have failed. Specific examples of when specialist input should be sought include: The presence of dementia is uncertain, the patient is young (<65), the dementia is rapidly progressive, motor symptoms are prominent, behavioral disorder is pronounced, the dementia is potentially reversible, or the care needs are beyond those usually required.

The assessment of dementia utilizes medical skills that are within the capabilities of all physicians. Some elements of the evaluation such as history taking, simple cognitive testing, and psychosocial assessment can be performed by allied professionals (nurses, psychologists, or social workers) who are specially trained.

In most cases, evaluation can be carried out by an interdisciplinary team. In this model, an allied health professional takes the history from the family and caregiver and performs a mental status exam, a neuropsychologist administers the neuropsychological assessment, and a physician performs a physical examination and comprehensive mental status exam and reviews the case with the other professionals. We believe such a model can be applied to any practice setting with the appropriate training and experience.

The physician who does not have such a team available should take the history, perform a physical examination and mental status examination of cognitive and noncognitive realms, and order appropriate laboratory studies. Indications for laboratory studies and referrals to a neuropsychologist and other professionals are discussed later on in this chapter.

What Processes Are Involved in a Dementia Assessment?

A comprehensive assessment is typically done in stages (Table 2.2).

The first stage involves the patient and one or more informants, requires 1–2 hours, and consists of the complete neuropsychiatric assessment (discussed below). The second stage consists of a family evaluation and is done only if the initial assessment confirms the diagnosis of dementia. It can be performed by a social worker or nurse and requires approximately 1 hour to complete. This, too, will be discussed below.

Table 2.2. Stages of a Comprehensive Dementia Evaluation

Stage 1
Neuropsychiatric assessment (directed by any trained physician)

Stage 2
Family assessment

Stage 3
Diagnostic tests

Stage 4
Conference discussion, diagnosis, and recommendations to patient, family, and others as appropriate

A series of diagnostic tests described later in this chapter should be obtained. These include laboratory studies, brain imaging studies, and neuropsychological testing. They are almost always done on an outpatient basis, but an inpatient assessment might be necessary if severe medical or behavioral problems are present. Finally, the whole picture is pulled together at a "Diagnostic and Recommendation Conference" where the interdisciplinary team meets with the patient and care providers to review the history and the results of assessment, to explain the diagnosis and prognosis, and to develop a treatment plan.

Each of these stages, including the initial assessment, has several purposes. Family and/or other informant involvement is crucial at several points but the patient and family should be evaluated separately to diminish patient embarrassment and allow family members to answer freely questions about the patient's history and current symptoms. Performing the entire assessment with patient and family together can be awkward and uncomfortable since the patient is being "talked about" as if she were not there. On rare occasions, patients will refuse to be seen alone. We sometimes call the family by telephone at another time to collect information and address concerns.

We typically start an assessment by meeting briefly with the patient and all family members who are present. We begin by stating that we will first meet with everyone, then talk with the patient and family separately, and conclude by meeting together to discuss the findings. Before separating the patient and family, we ask whether there are particular issues which should be discussed with everyone present. We specifically ask whether there are questions that the patient and family want addressed by the end of the evaluation. Occasionally the family will begin to give a full history at this point. If this happens we ask them to wait until later. The purpose of this brief joint meeting is to raise general issues that can be explored separately with both care provider and patient. Sometimes patients will say that they do not know why they are coming for an evaluation and do not want to be there. In this case, they can often be reassured that the evaluation will be relatively brief and that they will be returning home in an hour or two.

THE NEUROPSYCHIATRIC ASSESSMENT

The cornerstone of a comprehensive dementia evaluation is the neuropsychiatric assessment which is outlined in Table 2.3. The goal of this assessment is to obtain information that will enable the clinician to determine an initial impression, develop a differential diagnosis, and plan treatment. Selected sections of this evaluation are highlighted here.

Table 2.3. Outline of a Neuropsychiatric Assessment

1. *Identifying data:* age, marital status, race, sex, referral source

2. *Chief complaint:* including reason for referral and questions to be answered

3. *Family history:* vital status of parents, grandparents, siblings, and children; if deceased, age at death and cause; any members with psychiatric or neurological illness; pedigree

4. *Personal and social history:* where born, summary of early life experience, education, work history, marital state, living situation, leisure practices, religious faith, typical daily activities

5. *Current psychosocial environment:* living environment at present, care providers, financial issues, legal issues, use of community resources.

6. *Substance abuse:* use of cigarettes, alcohol, prescription, and over-the-counter medications; history of abuse or dependency on any of the above

7. *Medical history:* medical and surgical problems; active problems and their severity; review of systems, current medications, physicians and other health care providers involved in providing medical care

8. *Premorbid personality:* traits, predispositions, affect, activity, reactivity

9. *Neuropsychiatric history:* psychiatric symptoms or disorders, psychiatric assessments or treatments, seizures, head trauma, stroke, other neurologic disorders

10. *History of present illness:* onset date, course, features, rapidity, and pattern of change; systematic review of systems to include information on cognitive capacity, mental syndromes, unusual experiences, functional status, and behaviors

11. *Examinations:* physical, neurologic, cognitive, and mental status exam

12. *Laboratory evaluations:* brain imaging, laboratory studies, and other tests

Family history. A detailed family history of the grandparents, parents, siblings (brothers and sisters), and children is taken. This is best recorded as a pedigree on a genogram. An example is provided in Figure 2.1. A genogram helps the clinician and family ask questions about each relative and increases accuracy. This helps the clinician focus on family health history, which will aid in differential diagnosis, and on the current status of the family, which will identify potential and actual human resources available for the patient's care.

Personal history. The patient's personal background provides the data by which the whole case can be understood. In addition to allowing an estimation of premorbid functioning and cognitive reserve, the personal history illustrates the patient's life in a way that allows a clearer understanding of this individual and his or her response to illness. It also identifies interests and wishes, which in turn guide treatment planning. A sexual history should be obtained to assess for possible exposure to HIV risk factors.

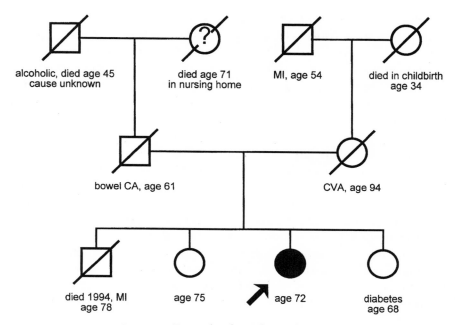

Figure 2.1. Example of a pedigree drawing.

Substance abuse history. It is important to be complete because several dependency-producing substances, including alcohol and benzodiazepines, impair cognition even at low doses.

Medical history and review of systems. This is essential. All patients should be asked about hypertension, diabetes, heart disease, cancer, lung disease, surgery and blood transfusions. Careful attention should be given to determining all medications taken in the last 6 months. Over-the-counter medicine such as aspirin and sleeping potions as well as herbs are important to note. Possible exposure, including occupational exposure, to toxins such as heavy metals (lead), organic solvents, and other chemicals should be determined.

Premorbid personality. This will provide a good picture of the patient's predispositions, character, temperament, and interests. It is important in understanding symptoms and in planning treatment and supportive care.

Neuropsychiatric history. Special attention is paid to a history suggestive of brain injury including trauma, transient ischemic attacks, stroke, paralysis, sensory loss, speech or language impairment, and tremor. A full psychiatric history is also taken including a history of mental symptoms such as depression, prior evaluation, or prior treatment, including hospitalization.

History of present illness. The examiner should identify the earliest symptoms and provide a chronological history up to the present using a detailed symptom checklist (Table 2.4). Family members and other informants play a major role in obtaining this part of the history. They should be asked specific questions about the functions and impairment listed in Table 2.4. In addition to helping with the differential diagnosis, this symptom checklist aides in the identification of target symptoms requiring treatment.

Cognitive and mental status examinations. Since the primary symptoms of dementia involve impairments in cognition, behavior, and function, a thorough mental status examination is a necessary part of the evaluation. Some clinicians believe the mental status examination is intrusive while others are concerned that it is insulting or too medical. Similar reluctance was reported years ago about taking a sexual history. Refusal is rare if the examiner believes it is an important part of the examination and tells this to the patient. It is helpful to assure the patient that this is part of the assessment for every person. Those who resist are almost always impaired in our experience. When individuals refuse to answer individual questions by saying, "That's a silly thing to ask" or "Of course I can do that," it is best to turn temporarily to another area of questioning such as the medical history and to repeat these questions later.

It is not uncommon for cognitively impaired patients to be reluctant to answer direct questions. Individuals who will not or cannot answer direct questions about cognition are more likely to answer questions asked in the course of a general conversation. For example, orientation to year can be determined during the life history review. "Where were you born? What year was that? Do you know what year it is now? How old does that make you?"

Resistance to the mental status examination can sometimes be overcome by the examiner's emphasizing that the assessment is being carried out to identify remaining abilities as well as impairments ("Let's see how well you do with this one") and by acknowledging that some questions are difficult. ("I'm going to ask you a more difficult one now. Let's see how good you are at math. Take 7 away from 100.") Sometimes it is useful to say that the information is being gathered for the benefit of the patient. ("I know this is hard, but if I know what you have problems with I'll be better able to help you.") There is a fine line between being supportive and being condescending, but helping a person over a difficult question is often reassuring. For example, if a person answers the question, "Do you know where we are now" with "I can't remember" and is upset, the examiner can be supportive by responding, "Well let me help you. Do you know what city are we in?" Even in the best of

Table 2.4. Symptom Checklist in the Evaluation of Dementia

Impaired Cognition	Impaired Function	Mood, Mental Phenomena	Behaviors	Drives
Memory	Cooking	Depression	Verbal abuse	Appetite poor
Language	Finances	Self-depreciating	Uncooperative	Weight loss
Orientation	Housekeeping	Somatic complaint	Physically aggressive	Excessive appetite
Writing/reading	Shopping	Crying spells	Sundowning	Hypersexuality
Calculating	Driving	Diurnal variation	Demands interaction	Hyposexuality
Recognizing	Hearing/sight	Withdrawn	Outbursts	Sleep poor
Attention/concentration	Dressing	Anxiety	Catastrophic	Sleeps a lot
Planning/organization	Mobility or falls	Fatigues easily	Noisy	Out of bed at night
Personality change	Bathing/grooming	Death, suicidal	Wandering	
Executing	Feeding	Disinterested	Hoarding/rummaging	
Social rules	Continence	Anhedonic	Sexual aggression	
		Energy level low	Intrusive	
		Apathetic		
		Panic		
		Labile		
		Irritable		
		Euphoria		
		Delusions		
		Illusions		
		Rapid speech		
		Hallucinations		
		Acute confusion		

hands, however, some individuals (perhaps 1%–2%) are unwilling to undergo this part of the assessment.

The mental status examination we recommend has seven major headings. An outline is presented in Table 2.5. It is not necessary to ask them all together. For example, some aspects of the mental status examination can be assessed during the general patient interview. Examples include appearance and behavior, talk, and mood. However, focused questions pertaining to these and other areas are usually neces-

---

Table 2.5. Parts of the Mental Status Examination

1. Appearance/Behavior

2. Talk
   Rate
   Rhythm
   Fluidity
   Spontaneity
   Latency
   Thought disorder

3. Mood and Affect
   Observed and reported stability, reactivity, and appropriateness
   Vital sense
   Self-attitude
   Thoughts of death, suicide, homicide

4. Perception
   Hallucinations
   Illusions

5. Content of Thought
   Delusions
   Obsessions
   Compulsions
   Phobias

6. Insight and Judgment

7. Cognition
   Consciousness
   Orientation
   Memory
   Praxis
   Language
   Abstraction
   Gnosis
   Knowledge
   Attention
   Calculation
   Executive Function

---

sary and it is useful for the examiner to have a specific outline in mind. This allows the clinician to check at the end of the evaluation and determine if all appropriate questions have been asked. It is also helpful to record the information obtained in a specific order because it allows the clinician to check for completeness and, more important, put the information together in a meaningful fashion. In addition, having the data in a specific order enables the clinician to present it to others in a comprehensive fashion.

The General Mental Status Examination

Appearance and behavior. First and foremost, practitioners are nonjudgmental observers who should record what they see and hear and avoid interpretation. Training and experience guide what the clinician considers relevant. Issues of note include whether patients recognize the clinician as a professional, whether they act in a manner consonant with their background, and whether they are well kempt in appearance. In general, the patients' approach to the examination reflects how they react in situations that are unusual or stressful.

The predominant demeanor of the patient during the assessment should be noted. Are they relaxed and calm, tense or distressed? Does the examiner have to work hard to put them at ease? Are they restless, slow moving, fidgety, or tremulous? Are there frequent, easily induced changes in mood or behavior? None of these is necessarily "abnormal" but each can be relevant for diagnosis and treatment.

Observing how patients are dressed is important. Are their clothes neat or do they seem disheveled, mismatched, misbuttoned, or dirty? Are they appropriate for the weather? Individuals who are reported to have always been neat and who come in with messy or stained clothes are probably having significant trouble not only with dressing but with other complex activities such as preparing meals and keeping house. These clues should raise concern about safety.

The description of behavior should also state whether patients are able to walk into the room unaided, require a wheelchair, use a cane, or are lying in bed. Do they have the stooped posture and flexed body habitus of a person with parkinsonism? Is there obvious weakness or does the person seem to neglect one side of the body? Are there rapid jerking movements? Do they appear fearful—for example, glancing around the room as if hearing someone talking? Do they seem disinterested, sad, or resistant? Did they become more or less cooperative as the assessment evolves?

Talk. Several aspects of the patients' talk (speech) should be assessed. First, speech should flow naturally (*fluency*) and spontaneously—that is, its speed should follow the examiner's. Speech should demonstrate appropriate rate, rhythm, and prosody (smoothness). The pragmatics of speech (appropriate use of facial expression and gestures in conversation) should be assessed.

Hesitant speech, in which word-finding difficulty is prominent, speech is telegraphic or without usual connecting words, and talking is frustrating to the patient, suggests a nonfluent (Broca) aphasia. Speaking a great deal but saying little that makes sense indicates a fluent (Wernicke) aphasia. Substituting one word for another, for example, calling a "watch" a "tie," or saying words that are combinations of other words ("time teller" for "watch") or totally new words ("when" for "watch")—all called *paraphasic errors*—also indicate a language disorder. Occasional difficulty finding words in the course of a conversation can be normal but repeated instances are not. Therefore, it is important to notice that such difficulties have occurred and to keep track of their frequency.

Second, are they able to *comprehend* questions and to *follow instructions*? An inability to do so in response to a normally spoken voice might be due to a hearing deficit but often indicates difficulty in comprehending spoken language (receptive aphasia). Do they ask for questions and instructions to be repeated? Do they seem to understand simple and straightforward questions but have difficulty with more complicated ones, even when asked with the same loudness of voice?

If words are *slurred* or incomprehensible, a disorder of the motor or production aspects of speech is likely. This points to damage of the neurological or oropharyngeal control mechanisms responsible for producing speech. In contrast, word-finding problems are indicative of an impairment of language processing.

The ability to control speech can be impaired. Hesitancy before answering questions and speaking very softly, slowly, and deliberately can indicate depression. Rapid speech that dominates the conversation and prevents the examiner from interrupting (pressure of speech) suggests hypomania or mania. If the content of speech does not flow logically, there might be evidence of tangentiality (answering questions well off the mark), circumstantiality (giving excessive detail), or derailment (having no clear "string" or line of thought). *Palilalic* speech, consisting of repetitive sounds such as "la la la," or words ("go go go"), or frequent perseveration (repetition) of words or phrases, indicates a severe language disorder.

Mood and affect. Clinicians sometimes distinguish between the terms *mood* and *affect* although there is not universal agreement on their definitions. It is best to describe both how patients feel in their own words (subjective mood) and how the examiner perceives their predominant mood to be (observed mood). It is always helpful to use quotations specifying the patients' exact words. Variations in mood during the course of the interview and examination should be described if they occur. The examiner should note if patients cry or laugh easily and if they are emotionally labile. Mood should reflect what the conversation is about; for example, when patients talk about someone's death they should appear sad. A lack of reactivity and evidence of "monotony" in mood should be noted. Irritability, anxiety, and emotional explosiveness or anger when confronted with a difficult task (a catastrophic reaction) are also important to report.

Vital Sense. This refers to patients' assessment of their energy level and whether it differs from their usual self-perception. Patients should be asked if they feel interested and energetic with regard to their usual activities, whether they derive enjoyment from usually enjoyed pleasure, whether their body feels well or sick, and whether they feel they would be able to sustain activity over time.

Self-attitude. This is a complicated construct that assesses how patients perceive their own capabilities and whether they believe these are different from their usual self-concept. Self-attitudes can be elevated with better than usual self-confidence and self-esteem or lower than usual with guilt, remorse, self-deprecation, self-blame, and feelings of incompetency and failure. Low self-attitude is often accompanied by hopelessness while elevated self-attitude often coexists with an inappropriately elevated and grandiosity. Fluctuations in self-attitude, especially those not linked to environmental events, might be indicative of a mood disorder. Even when dementia is present, the assessment of change in self-attitude is a particularly good way of determining the presence or absence of a mood disorder.

Assessment for thoughts of death, suicide, or homicide. Patients who can understand should be asked if they have thoughts about death, catastrophe, or disaster. Do they wish death upon themselves and, if so, why? Do they think they would be better off dead? Would they consider hurting themselves? If they would rather be dead but are not thinking of hurting themselves, what is stopping them? Are they angry with someone else? Are they thinking of hurting someone? What is the reason for this? What has prevented them from doing it thus far?

Perception. The examiner should investigate the presence of both hallucinations and illusions. *Hallucinations* are sensory perceptions without actual stimuli. They can occur in any of the five sensory modalities (hearing, sight, smell, taste and touch). Visual hallucinations are the most common in persons with dementia. The examiner should ask patients if they hear sounds or people or see things when nobody else is around or that others do not hear or see, whether there are peculiar or odd odors which they smell that others cannot, or if there has been a specific repetitive taste or sensation that has been upsetting. Hallucinations are distinguished from *illusions*. In the latter there is an actual stimulus which is misinterpreted or distorted; for example, seeing a face in the folds of the curtains, believing a lamp is an animal, or looking into a mirror and seeing the face of a stranger.

Thought content. This refers to ideas, beliefs, and explanations a person reports. Included under this heading is the presence of *delusions*. These are defined as ideas that appear to the examiner to be false, fixed (unshakable), and idiosyncratic (unique to that person). Delusions are common in persons with dementia, are often a source of distress to them and others, and can lead to problems in behavior. Common delusions in dementia include the belief that someone is coming into the house and stealing, that family members are taking money, or that a spouse is unfaithful. It is important to distinguish between delusions and ideas based on culture and background. One helpful way is to ask family, friends, and acquaintances whether they also believe what the patient believes. For example, the patient might have a religious belief which the examiner does not hold. If relatives have the same belief then it is unlikely to be a delusion and the most appropriate conclusion is that the difference between the examiner's and patient's perspective rests on culture rather than a disordered content of thought.

Obsessions, compulsions, and phobias are also surveyed. *Obsessions* are recurrent, intrusive *thoughts* that the subject perceives as his own and attempts to resist. They often concern trivial or foolish matters as described by the patient. Over time resistance may fade. Typical obsessions include preoccupation with cleanliness, orderliness, infestation, and disaster. *Compulsions* are repetitive *behaviors* that the person feels driven to perform, such as handwashing or touching the wall but which a person perceives as unreasonable and attempts to resist. Compulsions often occur in response to obsessions and are followed by a reduction in anxiety. *Phobias* are disproportionate fears of specific objects or situations. They should be distinguished from the fearfulness that arises in response to a delusion or depression. Although obsessions, compulsions, and phobias occur in patients with dementia they are usually manifestations of a psychiatric disorder which preceded the dementia.

Insight and judgment. *Insight* refers to a patient's awareness of cognitive or other deficits or of certain abnormal mental states. Insight is often impaired or lacking in dementia patients, especially in patients with one of the cortical dementias. This lack of awareness is a consequence of the underlying dementia rather than a psychological denial since it is uncommon in the subcortical dementias. The inability to perceive a deficit is called an anosagnosia. Insight is assessed by asking questions such as, "Do you think there is something wrong?" or specific questions relating to that individual's function, such as, "Is your memory functioning okay or are you having difficulty with it?" The lack of insight can explain what seems to be foolish, dangerous, or unusual behaviors, and more importantly, indicate ways in which physicians and other caregivers should best relate to the patient. For example, a severely impaired patient with poor insight is best not confronted with a diagnosis of a degenerative disorder such as Alzheimer disease because this could lead to brief distress without a clear benefit (since the patient cannot become aware that there is a deficit).

Judgment refers to a person's ability to assess a situation, consider the facts and issues, and draw an appropriate conclusion.

It can be assessed by asking questions about a health-related situation—for example, "If you had a serious health problem who would you talk to?" Judgment is also assessed from the history provided by the family and through the course of the interview by observing the way in which the patient approaches the examiner.

Elements of The Cognitive Mental Status Examination

Since cognitive impairment is the core feature of all dementias, every patient should undergo a thorough direct assessment of cognition. The extent of the cognitive assessment can vary, however, depending upon the purposes of the examiner and the setting. A neuropsychologist would be expected to carry out an in-depth extensive inventory of a person's cognitive abilities that would take several hours. A social worker, nurse, or physician reassessing a person with Alzheimer disease might use a brief, global assessment to monitor the patient's course.

The cognitive assessment should also be varied based on the patient's background. Individuals who have always been very bright or have depended on intellectual functions for their livelihood often need to be asked more complex questions to identify and assess cognitive deficits. For example, a bookkeeper should be able to do more complex math. Patients with other strengths should be tested in areas about which they are especially knowledgeable. Given the wide variability in premorbid ability and exposure, there is no single assessment instrument that is appropriate for all situations or all patients.

Nonetheless, it is useful to have a standard method of cognitive examination with which one starts and then modifies as appropriate for an individual patient. The most widely used standard cognitive examination is the MMSE developed by Folstein, Folstein and McHugh. The major strengths of this examination are its brevity and broad coverage of cognitive functions. Its chief limitations are an inability to identify very early dementia (called a *ceiling effect*), its dependence on language (resulting in very low scores in persons who have primary aphasia), and its inability to discriminate degree of impairment in severely impaired individuals (called a *floor effect*). As is the case with all cognitive tests, persons with low education do less well. Despite these limitations, the MMSE is a useful tool for assessing and following most individuals with dementia. It can also be used by the individual practitioner to follow "normal" individuals over time since a *sustained* drop of 3–4 points indicates a high likelihood of dementia. An occasional patient will "remember" items from a previous testing but this is rarely a problem in clinical settings. There are several methods used to score the MMSE. What is presented below is the version we most often use. Consistency of scoring is important so that an individual's performances can be compared over time and so that the capacities of different individuals can be compared and constrasted.

The Mini-Mental State Examination. The first half of the MMSE consists of items related to memory, attention, and concentration. The second half measures "cortical" functions. Items 1 and 2 measure *orientation* to time and place. Questions include, "Can you tell me where we are now?" and "What city and state are we in?" One point is given for each correct answer. When testing orientation to time (knowledge of the year, month, season, day of the week, and date) the first question asked may depend on whether, based on conversation, the person appears to have a significant impairment. If disorientation is likely, we often first ask if they know the month and introduce the questioning in a nonthreatening fashion—for example, "Have you been keeping up with the date? Do you know what month it is?" When a person is doing well, every question should be asked, even the year, since mildly impaired patients sometimes know the day and date but not the year.

Item 3 tests *registration*—that is, the ability to immediately repeat back items being committed to memory. This is the first part of *memory testing*. Three words are given to remember in the following manner: "I'd like to test your memory by asking you to remember three words. Please listen carefully and repeat the three words after me." We always choose the same three words for new patients. This not only has the benefit of preventing embarrassment should the examiner forget the words (or forget to write them down) but also teaches the examiner that normal individuals are able to repeat three words without difficulty unless they have a marked hearing deficit. This item is scored by counting the number of words the person is able to correctly repeat the *first* time. If a person misstates a word they do not receive a point for it. If they ask for the words to be repeated, the examiner should first ask them to repeat as many words as they do remember since the score for registration measures how many words an individual reports on the first try. The three words are repeated until the patient is able to say all three or it is clear that they cannot be said all at once.

Difficulty in registering the words can indicate a hearing problem or a language problem. If not previously alerted to the possibility of a hearing problem, the examiner should note this as a possibility and perform a hearing assessment at some point. Sometimes the examiner can raise his voice and find that the patient is still unable to respond to a command or question appropriately. Whispering words or commands in the patient's ear and having them listen to a watch or tuning fork are other forms of brief auditory testing.

The next item serves two functions. First it distracts the patient from reciting the three words just asked, and second it is a test of *attention* and *concentration*. An individual with an eighth-grade-or-higher education is asked to subtract 7 from 100 and then to continue subtracting 7 from the answer. This is called "serial sevens." If it is clear that the respondent has memorized answers from past times the subtraction is altered and they are asked instead to subtract beginning from 101 or 103. This is one item that many practitioners do not expect older persons to perform correctly. It is a good example of why it is important to have experience testing the normal elderly. Experience and research demonstrate that individuals with an eighth-grade education or better can perform serial sevens. The speed of performance may slow down with age so the examiner should be patient. An individual who is able to take 7 away from 100 correctly should be able to do all the subtractions. One point is scored for each correct subtraction even if the previous subtraction was incorrect (so "93, 87, 80, 73, 66" is given 4 points).

When individuals do not attempt the first subtraction (note: we do not say whether they *can* not or *will* not) or when they have less than an eighth-grade education they are asked to spell backwards a five-letter word with three consonants in a row (usually "world" or "spray" as a backup). To determine whether the person has the ability to spell the word, it is best to ask them to spell the word "world" or "spray" forward and then when they are finished, to spell it backward. For the occasional person who misspells the word forward their incorrect spelling in reverse is used as the correct sequence. When scoring backwards spelling, a point is given for each response which matches the correct position in the sequence, "d-l-r-o-w." For example, "d-l-o-r-w" would score 3 points while "d-r-o-l-w" and "l-r-d-o-w" would score 2.

After the distraction task patients are asked if they can remember any of the three words that they were asked to remember (recall). It is important to give individuals adequate time. Those in their 80s may take 30 seconds to recall all three words. One point is given for each word correctly recalled. The words must be *spontaneously* remembered to receive a point. For words that cannot be recalled (and thus scored as no points) the examiner might want to determine if giving a cue or hint or asking the patient to chose the correct word from a list of words, some of which were not in the original three, improves performance. These can provide useful information but are *not* scored on the MMSE. For example, the person who cannot benefit from cues will need more direct help in remembering than someone whose memory benefits from cuing. In giving cues, the clinician might start with a category, for example, "One was an animal." If they are still unable to remember, give them a choice, such as "Was it a puppy, pony, or kitten?" Because the MMSE does not have a set time interval after which items are recalled it is sometimes best to attempt a recall task with a 5-minute interval, particularly if the patient seems to have memory difficulty but recalls the items correctly the first time.

Several aspects of language are assessed in the MMSE. *Naming* is tested by asking the person to name two simple objects—for example, a pen and a watch. A point is given for each correct response. Visually impaired individuals can be asked to name a pencil and a key placed in their palm. Examiners might also want to assess naming in more depth by asking the patient to name less common objects, for example, a button, an eraser, a lapel, the stem of a watch, shoelaces, or the buckle of a belt. Points are not given on the examination for these words but repeated failures suggest a naming deficit. *Repetition* is assessed by testing the ability to repeat a specific phrase. The suggested MMSE phrase is, "No if's, and's, or but's." The phrase must be repeated exactly, including all the s's at the end of the words. The patient is allowed only one attempt. One point is given for a correct repetition. An alternate phrase is "Methodist, Protestant, Episcopal." These sentences are difficult for individuals of some ethnic backgrounds or for individuals for whom English is not native. If there is a question about this being a problem, the sentence, "Today is a (sunny) day in the month of (April — substituting the current weather and month)" can be used in its place. It is necessary that the patient say each and every word correctly. Repetition is an excellent screen for determining whether a person has any language problem. It requires intact comprehension, intact registration, and intact expression of language. Repetition can be adversely affected by hearing impairment. If this is present it should be noted since this can have important clinical and therapeutic implications. The next item addresses the ability to *read* a sentence *and carry out* the action. Reading the sentence "Close your eyes" is included in the MMSE. A person should be asked to read the sentence to themselves and then carry out the action. The print should be large so that it can be easily read by those with visual problems. Some patients are able to say the sentence but not carry out the action. A point is not given in this case.

Following a *three step command* requires that people comprehend that the examiner wants them to do something, that they can hear what is said, and that they are able to carry out the three distinct steps. This tests several cognitive abilities but is most indicative of the ability called *praxis*, defined as the ability to carry out learned motor movements. The three-step command on the MMSE asks the subject to take a piece of paper in the right hand, fold it in half, and then place it on the floor. A point is given for each step done correctly. The reliability of this item is surprising to some people. Patients who are able to do only one or two steps when first asked will usually be able to do only the same number of steps when asked to do them a second time.

Next, a person is asked to *write* a sentence spontaneously. One point is given if it is a complete sentence (with a subject, and a verb), if it is grammatically correct, and if it does not contain language errors. Some patients say they do not know what to write. In this instance we encourage them to "Write anything that comes to mind." When an individual is still not able to write a simple sentence, the examiner might suggest one—for example, "Today is a (warm or cold) day," changing the adjective depending on the temperature. However, a point is given only if patient *spontaneously* writes a complete, grammatically correct sentence. Finally, the patient is asked to *copy* a design with two five-sided interlocking shapes. A point is given if each figure has five sides and five angles and if the overlap is a four sided figure. This assesses *visuospatial function and praxis.*

The interpretation of an MMSE total score depends on the presence or absence of noncognitive impairments (e.g., blindness, dominant arm weakness) which might account for the loss of certain points, as well as on the person's estimated premorbid cognitive abilities, based, among other things, on his education and occupation. An MMSE score of below 24 is indicative of significant impairment. For blind individuals, a score of 27 is probably normal as they would be unable to complete three items due to blindness. In contrast, a score of 25 might be abnormal for a person with a high premorbid ability, such as an attorney or nuclear physicist.

The expanded cognitive examination. The MMSE adequately tests orientation, memory, praxis, language, attention, and calculation. However, there are other aspects of cognition (see Table 2.5) such as consciousness, fund of knowledge, and executive function which are not assessed well by the MMSE. Since successful performance on the MMSE does not necessarily indicate the absence of a dementia, particularly in persons who premorbidly were quite high functioning intellectually, a more in-depth cognitive examination is sometimes indicated. The discussion below gives examples of other important aspects of the examination.

Level of consciousness is assessed by evaluating the patient's ability to engage and focus on the examination without fluctuation or "waxing and waning." The presence of any limitation or fluctuation in attention might be indicative of delirium. Attention can be tested by having the patient repeat a sequence of numbers. Normally, about seven numbers can be repeated forward and backward.

A more in-depth examination of recent *memory* (or memorizing or memory for newly learned material) includes determining whether the patient can recall lists longer than three words or recall the second pair of words when given the first word of the pair. Testing for current events (e.g., what is in the news) is also a memory test. Almost every intact individual knows who the current president is, for example; the ability to name the previous four presidents also strongly suggests intact memory. An ability to name previous presidents or to name the current vicepresident should be interpreted in light of the patient's estimated premorbid abilities. *Remote memory* (or memory for previously learned material) refers to previously learned material such as events from one's personal life; important dates; and names of prior acquaintances, historical events, or personalities. It is tested by asking the patient about dates, people, and places they would be expected to know. Failure to know the names and ages of grandchildren is a likely indication of impairment, for example.

A more detailed assessment of *praxis, planning,* and *visuospatial* function includes asking the patient to draw a flowerpot or to draw a clock with the numbers in the correct place and the hands pointing at "10 minutes past 11." Assessments of ideomotor (cannot make believe they are using a tool or instrument) and ideational (can imitate an action only if they copy someone else) praxis include asking patients to demonstrate how people brush their teeth, comb their hair, button a button, or salute.

Testing *fund of knowledge* provides information about premorbid intellectual ability and current intellectual ability. Questions asked include ones concerning knowledge of recent news events, the functioning of certain equipment (such as a barometer), the color of a ruby, or the capitals of certain states or countries.

Abstraction is an element of cognitive function that can be tested through proverb interpretation and the ability to identify similarities and differences. The interpretation of proverbs requires intact language skills but is primarily a measure of abstraction. Abstraction is strongly influenced by cultural factors. Thus, proverbs must be in the cultural repertoire of the patient to be appropriate. When testing this, it is common to start with an easily interpretable proverb such as, "Don't cry over spilled milk." ("What's done is done.") A second, more difficult proverb, is, "People who live in glass houses shouldn't throw stones," ("Don't criticize others if you also have faults.") Finally, another proverb used is, "A stitch in time saves nine." ("Don't put things off.") A difficult proverb that is unfamiliar to most individuals but that usually can be interpreted by individuals with intact normal intelligence is, "The tongue is the enemy of the neck." ("Don't talk too much.")

The ability to abstract can also be tested by asking individuals how an apple and orange are alike. The correct response is, "They both are fruit." If an incorrect answer such as "They are both round" is given, the examiner should say "And they're both fruit. Now try this one." Subsequently, more difficult pairs of items are given, such as a hammer and a saw (tools), a table and a chair (furniture), a bicycle and an airplane (means of transportation), or a bird and a tree (both alive). The ability to abstract is also tested by asking the difference between a river and canal (natural vs. man-made) or a dwarf and a child (a child will grow tall).

Tests that require the ability to focus attention and switch sets (concepts) in rapid succession, sometimes referred to as *executive function*, should be considered, particularly when frontal lobe impairment is possible. Three tests are commonly used in this regard. The first is a verbal form of the Trail Making Test. The test is introduced by saying, "I'm going to ask you to alternate numbers with letters. Please complete the sequence. 1A, 2B, keep going." This requires the ability to recite the alphabet and to count to 13. The examiner keeps track of the patient's responses and corrects them as needed. For example, the patient might say 1A, 2B, 3C, 4D, 5F, in which case the examiner would say "5-E, keep going." If the patient reverses the sequence, as in "1-A, 2-B, C-3, 4-D", no correction or penalty is applied. Two minutes are allowed for the patient to go all the way to 13-M. The examiner keeps track of time. Taking more than 60 seconds or making three or more errors indicates impairment.

A second test of executive function is the Luria Hand-Sequencing Test, in which the patient is asked to mimic or copy a sequence of hand movements done by the examiner: The examiner demonstrates a series of three hand positions, or movements, for example, an open palm, a fist, and scissor fingers. After each set of three hand positions the patient is asked to copy the exact sequence. Five sets of three positions are given. Most well elderly patients are able to successfully copy four or five in the absence of impairment. Younger persons can do better.

The final test is referred to as the Go–No Go Test. In this the examiner gives the instruction, "I am going to tap on the table with my fist. If I tap once I want you to respond by tapping twice. If I tap twice I want you to respond by not tapping at all." Ten trials are given. Most well elderly respondents can successfully complete six or seven of 10; younger persons can do better, often a perfect 10.

Use of Standardized Scales to Supplement Assessment

The process of assessment is often complemented by the use of a limited number of standardized scales that assess different domains. The rating of these scales allows the clinician to summarize and organize a complex case by reference to a set of numbers. This is useful in communicating information about severity to other caregivers, provides an objective means of charting course over time, and helps assess response to interventions.

Many scales have been developed for rating different features of dementia. We favor the use of scales that are simple to administer, have been shown to be reliable, and have broad coverage. The domains that are important to consider are cognition, mood, behavioral disturbances, and daily living activities (both instrumental and basic).

To rate cognition in early and moderately advanced stages we recommend the MMSE. For late-stage patients we recommend the Severe Impairment Rating Scale (SIRS). To rate depression we recommend the Cornell Scale for Depression in Dementia (CSDD). To rate dependency on caregivers and to assist in level of care decisions, the Psychogeriatric Dependency Rating Scale-Behavior (PGDRS) subscale is preferred. To rate instrumental activities of daily living we recommend The IADL (Lawton and Brady, 1988), and to rate activities of daily living the PGDRS-Physical subscale. To rate behavioral disturbance in dementia, we favor the Neuropsychiatric Inventory (NPI). References for these scales are included at the end of this book.

THE FAMILY ASSESSMENT

The importance of an evaluation of the patient's family and personal environment cannot be overemphasized. The family has been described as "the lifeline of the patient." Their well-being is essential to the patient's status and the family is appropriately considered a partner in care. As professionals embark on the care of the patient and family it must be remembered that the provision of a diagnosis and treatment recommendations will aid the family in the years ahead but must be supplemented by the many other approaches discussed in this book. Data on the family that are collected around the time of the initial contact can be crucial for understanding the family's needs.

Table 2.6 lists the elements important to the family and their assessment. The family's well being is best monitored over time by revisiting these areas at intervals of no longer than 6 months. Although family assessment is frequently provided by social workers it can be accomplished by other health care providers as long as the information gathered is systematically collected. Construction of a family genogram is one effective way to gather these data. An example is in Figure 2.1.

The assessment of the patient's functioning within the family should cover the following particular topics: knowledge of how the patient's needs and wants are provided for; the way in which the patient spends his (her) time; the extent to which family and/or care providers have insight into the patient's condition and its prognosis; the extent to which care-providers require help in caring for the patient; and the resources family caregivers have available to provide help.

Through the psychosocial assessment the clinician will develop an understanding of the patient's immediate environment, day-to-day functioning, and resources. This will add to the intervention problem list and lay the groundwork for developing appropriate long-term supportive care for the patient and family (see Chapters 7 and 8).

Table 2.6. Assessment Domains for the Family Evaluation

1. Family members, their roles, frequency of interaction

2. Health status of care providers

3. Financial status of care providers

4. Spiritual beliefs

5. Knowledge about dementing illnesses

6. Other responsibilities, including work and other dependents, such as children or other ill relatives

DIFFERENTIAL DIAGNOSIS AND WORKUP
OF DEMENTIA

After completing the assessment discussed in the beginning of this chapter, the clinician is faced with the task of making sense of the information. Doing so has two purposes—diagnosing the cause of the dementia and developing a care plan. A list of possible diagnoses, called the *differential diagnosis,* is made, and this clarifies what other information is needed.

The goals of differential diagnosis are formulation, classification, and determination of cause. This process is best understood in a series of sequential steps (outlined in Figure 2.2) to which we refer throughout the remainder of this chapter.

In the *formulation,* the clinician organizes the history, physical examination, mental status examination, and laboratory studies in a coherent and systematic fashion. The first step is to decide whether dementia is present or absent. If cognitive impairment is absent (in which case dementia is absent) the differential diagnosis typically involves disorders such as depression, schizophrenia, factitious disorder, or a neurologic disorder that spares cognition. If cognitive impairment is present then the clinician must decide if the *clinical* definition of dementia is met (i.e, a global decline in cognitive capacity in clear consciousness). If cognitive impairment is present but dementia is not, then another diagnosis such as amnestic disorder, aphasia, mild cognitive disorder, or age-associated memory impairment should be considered. If the clinician is still uncertain about the presence or absence of dementia after the initial assessment, then long term follow-up will be necessary to determine whether dementia is present. Uncertainty is most common when the patient was highly functioning premorbidly and is only mildly impaired, when the clinician is not persuaded that the patient's current functioning represents a decline, or when the patient is very old. Neuropsychological testing, a series of standardized and normed tests of cognitive function performed by a specially trained clinician, can be an invaluable tool in the evaluation of dementia. Referral for testing is indicated when there is cognitive impairment but it is not clear if it is severe enough to be a dementia, when the impairment could be accounted for by advanced age, when there is dementia but there is uncertainty about its cause, or when there is a need to differentiate dementia from depression or schizophrenia.

If the clinician decides that dementia is present, then the next step is the *classification* of the syndrome according to its cognitive features (cortical, subcortical, mixed), severity (mild, moderate, severe) noncognitive features (behavior, mood), motor disturbances, and severity of

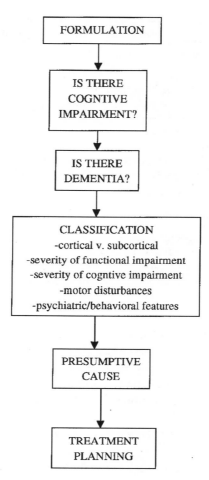

Figure 2.2. Flow diagram for the differential diagnosis in a case of suspected dementia.

impairments in functioning. This classification lays the foundation for determining etiology and directing treatment. Tables 1.2, 1.4, and 1.5 will assist in this classification.

The final step in *differential diagnosis* is a determination of likely cause. Table 1.3 compares a list of common causes of dementia. The presumptive cause is arrived at by matching the patient's history, signs, and symptoms with known disorders (see Chapters 3 and 4). Further clinical and historical data as well as laboratory, imaging or neuropsychological testing may be needed to determine a presumptive cause.

Table 2.7 lists laboratory investigations to consider for all patients with dementia. Some should be ordered in all cases. Brain imaging

Table 2.7. Laboratory Investigations for
the Evaluation of Dementia Syndromes

Urinalysis and Microscopy

Blood Tests
    Complete blood count
    Serum electrolytes, including magnesium
    Serum chemistries, including liver tests
    Thyroid testing
    B_{12}
    *Erythrocyte sedimentation rate
    Serologic tests for syphilis (or similar)

*Chest X-rays

*Electrocardiogram

*Toxicology screens
    Urine toxicology
    Serum toxicology (alcohol, salicylates, other)

*To be considered; not universally needed.

should be considered in all cases but is not necessary in all cases. If the dementia is longstanding (more than 3 years) or very advanced, imaging may not be necessary. If brain imaging is conducted, computed tomography (CT) is typically adequate. Magnetic resonance imaging (MRI), single photon emission computed tomography (SPECT), or positron emission tomography (PET) should be ordered to rule specific causes in or out (e.g., MRI for stroke or tumor, SPECT/PET to look for focal blood flow declines).

When the clinical circumstances, history, or examination indicates, that a *specific* cause might be present for which a specific diagnostic test is available (Table 2.8), it should be ordered.

The process of differential diagnosis (Figure 2.2) is a "top-down" process in which the clinical phenomena, both signs and symptoms, first determine the presence or absence of the syndrome of dementia and then direct the classification of the syndrome into recognizable patterns. Because it is assumed that in all cases of dementia there is an underlying disease of the brain, and since in most cases the clinical pattern correlates well with findings at autopsy, knowledge and understanding of the clinical syndrome are important. However, clinicians should not lose sight of the fact that in a sizable number of cases, perhaps 15–20%, the clinical presentation of dementia is "atypical"—that is, it does not follow a recognizable pattern and therefore the pathologic cause is less certain.

Table 2.8. Second Stage Laboratory Investigations

Test	Indication
Electroencephalogram(EEG)	Possible seizures; Creutzfeld-Jakob disease
Lumbar puncture	Onset of dementia <6 months; dementia rapidly progressive
Heavy metal screen	History of potential exposure
HIV test	History of potential exposure
Lyme disease titer	History of exposure and compatible clinical picture
Ceruloplasmin, arylsulfatase, electrophoresis	Wilson disease, metachromatic leucodystrophy, multiple myeloma
Slit lamp exam	History and exam suggest Wilson disease
Apolipoprotein E testing	Need to increase likelihood that AD diagnosis is correct
Genetic testing for Alzheimer genes or other dementia genes	Family history is strong and confirmation clinically necessary

We do not favor classifying dementia as reversible and irreversible, however. First, even when a dementia for which there is a specific treatment is diagnosed, it often does not fully respond to treatment, particularly if it has been present for more than several months. Second, many of the treatments that are available now and will become available in the near future will lead to partial or transient improvement, but not full recovery, in most patients with dementia.

3

Diseases Typically Causing a Cortical Pattern Dementia

One of the major themes of this book is that making a specific diagnosis of the cause of dementia is important because it conveys important knowledge about prognosis and treatment. Many disease processes lead to dementia and they differ substantially in what parts of the brain they affect and in their symptoms. For most of the diseases discussed, dementia is universally present. However, for a several, such as multiple sclerosis, dementia is not inevitable. Table 1.3 lists some of the 100 or so diseases associated with the clinical syndrome of dementia. Only the more common conditions and those that make important teaching points will be discussed in detail.

Diseases typically associated with cortical syndromes are discussed in this chapter. Diseases typically causing subcortical or mixed dementia syndromes are discussed in Chapter 4. For each disease, three areas are reviewed:

The clinical picture of the dementia syndrome associated with that disease, including prominent cognitive abnormalities, the associated noncognitive behavioral disorders, other common neurologic features, and the course and prognosis of the disease.

Epidemiology, including population prevalence (number of cases in the population), incidence (number of *new* cases in a given time period), and known risk factors.

Pathology (structural brain abnormalities) and *etiology* (cause) of the disease process. The focus is on the mechanism of brain injury associated with each disease process and how this mechanism leads to a specific dementia syndrome.

ALZHEIMER DISEASE

Clinical Picture

Alzheimer disease (AD) is defined clinically by the criteria (from McKhann, et al., 1984) listed in Table 3.1. Its earliest symptoms are often recognized only in retrospect because it has an insidious onset and is slowly progressive. The dementia of AD is a classic cortical dementia with impairments in memory (amnesia), coordination/dexterity (apraxia), language (aphasia), and perception (agnosia). Roughly speaking, the progression of the AD dementia is broken down into three clinical stages, each lasting 3 years on average. In the first stage, memory impairment predominates. In some individuals, personality changes occur as well. Impairment in IADL are present but ADL impairment is absent or minimal. In the second stage, patients develop significant impairments in language; in the ability to do everyday activities; and in recognition of people, places, and situations. Functioning becomes impaired to the point that they can no longer carry out unsupervised instrumental daily activities such as shopping, keeping with up bills, or cooking. In the third stage the impairments in memory, communication, and praxis and recognizing become severe. Impairments in basic capacities, such as walking and toileting, develop. As a result patients need considerable help with basic daily activities such as bathing, dressing, and mobility. Most patients in the third stage are fully dependent on others for basic daily activities.

Patients with AD frequently suffer from a variety of noncognitive behavioral disorders. Delusions, hallucinations, sleep disturbance, overactivity/aggression/agitation, and depression are most common. Delusions and misinterpretations occur in 30%–40% of patients with Alzheimer disease at some point in the illness. Ten to 25% experience an hallucination. These are most often visual, but auditory hallucinations also occur and can be distressing. The delusions and the hallucina-

Table 3.1. Criteria for Probable
Alzheimer's Disease

A. Dementia
   Decline on examination and objective testing
   Deficits in two or more areas of cognition

B. Gradual Progression

C. Level of Consciousness Intact

D. Onset after Age 40

E. No Other Cause after Workup

tions differ from those seen in schizophrenia. In AD the delusions are fairly circumscribed—that is, not very elaborate—for example, the belief that someone is stealing their money. It is rare for patients to offer complex explanations for how they know this and why it is occurring. Delusions and hallucinations can lead patients to troubling behaviors such as striking out at others, barricading in a room, hiding things, or refusing to eat.

The reported rates of depression in AD vary widely. In several studies in which patients have been evaluated thoroughly, 20%–25% were found to have depressive symptoms. Depression can lead to mental suffering, striking out, weight loss, and social disinterest.

A variety of problem behaviors develop in the middle and late stages of AD, but no widely accepted classification system has been developed. We group them according to their phenomenology (symptomatology) and by assumptions about the mechanisms which cause them. Added together, noncognitive symptoms afflict as many as 60% of patients with AD. However, since most of the data in this estimate comes from university-based outpatient clinics and nursing homes, it may be biased.

In the early stages of Alzheimer disease, neurologic symptoms are limited to the cognitive abnormalities. In the third stage, hyperreflexia, apractic gait, and frontal release signs (grasp and snout reflexes) develop. Some patients develop parkinsonian symptoms. Sudden jerking movements of limbs, trunk, or head, called *myoclonus,* occur in 15% of patients, and seizures occur in 10%. Difficulty walking due to gait apraxia and poor balance is common and fine motor coordination becomes progressively impaired. In the very late stages patients often become incontinent and immobile and develop problems with swallowing. In the preterminal stages many patients become bed-bound. Marked rigidity (stiffness) is common, as is diffuse hyperreflexia, spasticity, and inability to swallow.

Alzheimer disease lasts 8–10 years on average but cases as brief as 2 years and as long as 22 years have been reported and confirmed pathologically. For many patients the diagnosis is not made until a person has had symptoms for 2–3 years. The confidence in the clinical diagnosis based on the criteria in Table 3.1 is high. Over 90% of patients who meet these criteria are found to have the characteristic brain changes of the disease at autopsy. Decline is usually steady, and for most individuals the rate seems to stay consistent, but the rate of progression can vary. Some studies suggest an acceleration of the decline in the middle stage and slower declines early and late, but this may be due to the way decline is measured and to the fact that certain impairments such as language disorder are more impairing.

Epidemiology

The prevalence of Alzheimer disease (AD) is age-dependent. In the United States, 3%–5% of persons 65 years of age or older are estimated to suffer from Alzheimer disease. This number increases to 10%–15% for persons 75 years of age or older and to 20%–25% for persons 85 years of age or older. The estimates are consistent across almost all racial and cultural groups. The incidence of AD at age 65 is around 0.25% per year. This doubles every 5 years so that incidence is 1% per year at age 75 and approaches 4% per year at age 85.

Alzheimer disease is always associated with a dementia if one requires both the clinical syndrome and the brain pathology to make the diagnosis. However, some individuals are found at autopsy to have the pathology of Alzheimer disease without having manifested symptoms of a dementia syndrome. Since the pathology precedes the clinical syndrome, it is likely that all individuals who develop the pathology and live long enough will develop dementia, but this hypothesis cannot be tested at present.

Pathology and Etiology

The pathology of Alzheimer disease has two prominent features, both described by Dr. Alois Alzheimer in 1906–1907. First are extracellular accumulations called *neuritic* or *senile plaques*. These contain a protein predominantly consisting of beta-amyloid that is the breakdown product of a protein present in all nerve cell (neuron) membranes known as the *amyloid precursor protein* (APP). The way in which APP becomes beta-amyloid is not known. Under the microscope this protein stains in a characteristic pattern.

The second element of the brain pathology is the intracellular *neurofibrillary tangle*. This, too, is a protein, made up predominantly of hyperphosphorylated tau protein. This protein links together pieces of the cell microtubules that make up the cytoskeleton or skeleton of the cell. The precise ways in which neuritic tangles develop are also not known.

Another important finding in the pathology of AD is widespread loss of neurons. In the early stages of the disease, this is most prominent in the entorhinal and hippocampal areas of the temporal lobes. As the disease progresses, it spreads throughout the temporal and into the parietal regions. Cell loss is also found to varying degrees in the frontal lobes, subcortical structures such as the nucleus basalis of Meynert (the main source of brain acetylcholine), and deeper structures such as the locus ceruleus (the source of most brain norepinephrine) and the raphe nuclei (the source of most brain serotonin). This widespread loss of neurons accounts for the atrophied or shrunken appearance of the brain at autopsy.

The distribution of neuropathology helps explain the clinical syndrome. Neuritic plaques and neurofibrillary tangles in the hippocampus and entorhinal cortex are responsible for impaired memory. Temporal lobe pathology explains the prominence of language disorder while cell loss in the parietal lobes leads to visuoperceptual impairments. Loss of neurons occurring in subcortical nuclei such as the locus ceruleus and raphe nuclei may lead to hallucinations, delusions, and impaired regulation of mood.

The cause of the neuropathology and the mechanism by which it spreads are not yet known. Heredity plays an important role in the causation of the disease. About 5–10% of cases are transmitted as an autosomal dominant, with 50% of cases in each subsequent generation affected. Genes on chromosomes 21 (the APP gene), 1 (the presenilin-2 gene), and 14 (the presenilin-1 gene) have been implicated in the causation of AD in these familial cases. In addition, two other genes, on chromosome 19 (the apolopoprotein E gene) and on chromosome 12 (the alpha-2M gene), appear to increase the risk of developing AD and to affect the age of onset of AD. There are probably other genes involved in the development of AD.

In terms of the ways in which the pathology of AD develops, there are probably primary and secondary processes. It is not clear whether cell death initiates the process or if some other process initiates a cascade that leads to cell death secondarily. The death of neurons leads to the loss of neurotransmitter release, which in turn is associated with the development of specific symptoms. For example, the loss of acetylcholine is thought to lead to memory loss and perhaps other cognitive impairments. Loss of the neurotransmitters norepinephrine, dopamine, somatostatin, and serotonin is probably linked to the development of other specific cognitive and noncognitive symptoms.

FRONTOTEMPORAL DEGENERATION

A group of dementias in which there is variable degeneration of the frontal and temporal lobes is now referred to as *frontotemporal dementia* (FTD). These have been referred to by a variety of different names, including "dementia lacking distinctive histological features," "dementia of the frontal lobe type," "frontal lobe dementia," "frontal lobe degeneration," "lobar atrophy," and "Pick's disease." These conditions are grouped together because of their similar clinical picture and similarities in their neuropathology.

Clinical Picture

FTD usually begins with changes in personality, executive function, and behavior. Executive function refers to a set of capacities required to abstract; to follow social rules; to be mentally flexible; and to initiate, sustain, and stop behavior. Apathy, disinhibition, intrusiveness, explosiveness, irritability, and assaultiveness are common early manifestations of FTD. Depression, delusions, and hallucinations are relatively infrequent. Language disorders can occur early because the temporal lobes are often involved. Amnesia, aphasia, apraxia, and agnosia often develop within several years but are often less prominent than in AD. The motor dysfunction generally develops later in the disease and consists of slowness and rigidity, but gait disorder can be an early manifestation. Falls are frequent as a result. The average age of onset is 54 and average age of death is 64—that is, younger than for AD.

Diagnostic criteria for FTD are found in Table 3.2. These clinical criteria have not been linked to autopsy diagnosis, and their sensitivity and specificity for autopsy diagnosis are not known.

Four subtypes of FTD have been proposed:

In the frontal lobe type, disinhibition and poor insight are the earliest manifestations. Memory loss, rigidity, and dysarthria develop in the middle stage, followed by withdrawal, apathy, aphasia, and amimia (lack of spontaneity). The average duration is 5–7 years.

In the thalamostriatal type, personality changes and extrapyramidal motor symptoms such as rigidity and slowness occur early. Apathy and disinhibition are less common. The thalamostriatal type progresses more slowly, typically lasting 7–10 years.

Patients with the motor neuron type develop the spinal cord pathology and clinical symptoms of amyotrophic lateral sclerosis (ALS), or Lou Gehrig's disease, in addition to the characteristic brain pathology. Language and memory disorder occur early along with the frontal lobe symptoms. Duration is typically 2–4 years.

The asymmetric type resembles the frontal lobe type except that the condition localizes to the dominant temporoparietal area. Language disorder predominates if the dominant (almost always left) hemisphere is involved and visuospatial symptoms if the nondominant hemisphere is more involved. Duration is 2–4 years.

Epidemiology

The population prevalence of FTD is not known. Autopsy studies report its prevalence at 3% for all patients with dementia and 10% for patients with dementia who die before age 70. The disease has been re-

Table 3.2 Criteria for Frontotemporal Degeneration

A. Progressive Personality Change and Breakdown in Social Conduct
    Restless, distractible, disinhibited, OR apathetic, slowed, amotivated
    Hypochondriasis with bizarre complaints
    Stereotyped behavior
    Echolalia and perseveration
    Variable memory disturbance

B. Normal Neurologic Examination
    May have frontal release signs

C. Supportive Features
    Family history of dementia
    Reduced frontal lobe blood flow on functional imaging
    Normal EEG

ported throughout the world. It appears to have a substantial familial aggregation which may follow an autosomal dominant pattern.

Pathology and Etiology

Neuronal loss, astrocytosis (increased numbers of brain cells called *astrocytes*), and vacuolization (development of balloon-like areas) of the superficial layers of the frontal and temporal cortices are common to all forms of FTD. The subtypes are distinguished pathologically by variable involvement of subcortical and limbic structures. The frontal lobe subtype has less subcortical involvement, whereas in the thalamostriatal subtype there is prominent loss of neurons in multiple subcortical nuclei. In the motor neuron type there is loss of brain stem and spinal cord hypoglossal nucleus cells and anterior motor neurons. The asymmetric type has pathologic features similar to the frontal lobe type, but the dominant hemisphere (usually the left) is most affected. In some cases, characteristic abnormal inclusions called *Pick bodies* are found in the nuclei of dying neurons. In such instances the pathologic diagnosis of Pick disease is made. Recent research has indicated that FTD may be a heritable disease with an autosomal dominant inheritance, linked to the gene on chromosome 17, which codes for the tau protein.

DISSEMINATED LEWY BODY DISEASE

Clinical Picture

Dementia due to disseminated Lewy body disease (LBD) has been described in recent years. In addition to the impairments of memory, language, and praxis that are seen in cortical dementia, mild parkinsonism (resulting in falls), hallucinations, and delusions are present early in the course. Cognitive impairment can fluctuate over time so that days of moderate impairment alternate with nearly normal functioning. This fluctuation in conjunction with falls and the noncognitive psychopathology are central to making the diagnosis. At least 50% of patients have complex visual hallucinations and/or paranoid delusions. Auditory hallucinations occur in 15%. Depression is present in 40% of individuals.

Motor disorder is prevalent early in LBD, primarily manifested as parkinsonism (rigidity, slowed movements, and poor balance). Tremor is rare. Whenever parkinsonian symptoms and cognitive impairments characteristic of cortical dementia are present at the onset of a dementia, LBD should be strongly considered. Up to 40% of patients experience unexplained falls by the time they present to clinicians. As the disease progresses, the parkinsonian signs become more prevalent, occurring in more than 50% of patients. Neuroleptic drugs can cause a worsening of parkinsonism and lead to marked rigidity, tremor, postural instability, and gait disturbance even at low doses.

LBD appears to evolve in stages but good data are lacking. The earliest period consists of episodes of forgetfulness, lapses of concentration, periods of gait instability, and depression. Functional impairments are uncommon at this stage.

In the second stage, which often coincides with presentation for evaluation, the cognitive impairments continue to fluctuate but problems become frequent at night, perhaps due to distressing visual hallucinations, auditory hallucinations, and paranoid delusions. Extrapyramidal symptomatology leads to frequent falls. EEG abnormalities consisting of anterior temporal lobe theta and delta activity, often with sharp components and occasionally with marked lateral asymmetry, can be seen.

The third stage of LBD is characterized by a rather sudden acceleration of cognitive decline, delusions, hallucinations, and behavioral disturbance. The decline of the patient is fairly dramatic. Death may occur within months, typically due to aspiration. During this terminal phase patients can remain behaviorally disturbed with shouting, aggression, and delirium-like spells.

LBD shares similarities with both Parkinson disease and Alzheimer disease, but it can be distinguished from them both clinically and pathologically. Several sets of operational criteria have been proposed. Those of the group at Newcastle-Upon-Tyne in England are presented in Table 3.3. These have a good sensitivity (95%) and adequate specificity (82%) based on pathologic confirmation.

Age of onset of LBD is similar to Alzheimer disease; the median age

Table 3.3. Criteria for Disseminated Lewy Body Disease

A. Fluctuating Cognitive Impairment
   Memory and one other area affected
   Episodic confusion followed by lucid intervals

B. One of the Following
   Visual or auditory hallucinations, paranoid delusions
   Mild extrapyramidal symptoms or neuroleptic sensitivity
   Unexplained falls, transient clouding or loss of consciousness

C. *A* and *B* Sustained over a Period of Months

D. No Other Cause after Workup

E. No Evidence of Vascular Dementia

is in the early to mid-70s. Noncognitive symptoms occur earlier in the course of LBD than in Alzheimer disease. Duration of illness is shorter than for Alzheimer, ranging from 3 to 8 years.

Epidemiology

Since LBD has only recently been recognized as a distinct entity, precise epidemiologic data are not available. Between 5% and 18% of patients coming to autopsy suffer from LBD. Extrapolation of estimates for dementia suggest that perhaps 0.5%–1% of persons over 65 suffer from this disease. Although there appears to be a predominance of men suffering from this condition, this finding is controversial.

Pathology and Etiology

The hallmark pathology of the LBD is the Lewy (pronounced loowee in the United States and levee in Europe) body, an intracellular inclusion body. Lewy bodies were first described early in the century by a student of Alois Alzheimer, and for much of the 20th century were believed to occur primarily in Parkinson disease in the substantia nigra. In LBD, Lewy bodies are seen outside the substantia nigra in the cortex. Lewy bodies are relatively dense in the brain stem and in the entorhinal cortex and other areas of the temporal lobes. The parietal and frontal cortices exhibit lower counts of Lewy bodies. Lewy bodies are rare in the occipital cortices.

In some cases of LBD, senile plaques are common and reach levels similar to those seen in Alzheimer disease. However, few cases have sufficient numbers of neurofibrillary tangles to meet the criterion for Alzheimer disease. This has led some authors to suggest that there are two types of LBD, one called the *Lewy body variant of AD* and the other *LBD,* a distinct disease. Further studies are needed to clarify this.

Cholinergic activity is reduced in LBD, especially in the temporal, frontal, and parietal cortices. Loss of cholinergic function in the parietal cortex parallels impairments on mental tests of cognition. Cholinergic neuron counts have been found to be lower in hallucinating than non-hallucinating patients with LBD. This suggests that the cholinergic deficiency may play a role in the development of hallucinations.

Neuronal cell loss parallels the distribution of Lewy bodies just as the presence of plaques and tangles parallels cell loss in AD. Direct neuropathologic comparisons between Alzheimer disease, Parkinson disease, and senile dementia of the Lewy body type suggest that the qualitative aspects of the LBD pathology (i.e., the Lewy bodies) mostly resemble those of Parkinson disease although the distribution of this pathology resembles that of Alzheimer disease (that is, it is widely distributed in the brain).

The risk of developing a dementing disorder in the context of LBD is unknown although it is likely to be very high. No autopsy series have documented the presence of the LBD pathology in the absence of the clinical syndrome of dementia.

There is a correlation between the pathology in the temporal lobes and the hallucinatory syndrome and an association between the pathology in the parietal lobes and the severity of cognitive impairment. The unique clinical picture can be partly understood by the distribution of neuropathology, but much more work needs to be done to prove this.

THE PRION DEMENTIAS

Clinical Picture

This is a group of rare brain diseases first described in 1921. Presently, two forms of the disease have been associated with dementia, a sporadic (nonfamilial) form referred to as *Creutzfeld-Jakob disease* (CJD) and a familial (heritable) type referred to as *Gerstman-Straussler-Scheinker syndrome* (GSS) which follows an autosomal dominant pattern of transmission.

Early symptoms of prion dementia include executive dysfunction, aphasia, apraxia and amnesia. Progression is rapid and change can be observed over a period of several weeks. Motor disorders also occur early. These include myoclonus (brief, quick muscle jerks), spasticity, and ataxia.

The age of onset of the prion dementias is usually after age 55. Both sexes appear to be affected equally. There is some evidence that brain trauma might advance the age of onset of the disease. In nonfamilial cases the disease has a rapid onset and course, leading to death within

12–18 months, although longer durations of up to 5–6 years have been reported. The genetic forms of prion dementia are less malignant and run a more protracted course, particularly in women. The onset is usually characterized by personality change and disinhibition gradually followed by the four A's of cortical dementia.

A new form of CJD has emerged in Europe that typically begins between ages 20 and 40, presents with psychiatric symptoms and ataxia, and progresses in a fashion similar to the nonfamilial disorder. There is speculation that this is a human form of bovine spongiform encephalopathy (BSE), or "mad cow disease," but the link has not been proven.

Although systematic study is limited, noncognitive behavioral disorders such as depression, mania, delusions, and hallucinations are relatively rare in the nonfamilial form but common in the familial younger-onset form. Problem behaviors such as agitation and irritability may be more frequent but their prevalence is unknown.

At onset the diagnosis of prion dementia can be difficult, but the rapid progression and early myoclonus are suggestive. The EEG often shows generalized, repetitive triphasic complexes with virtual abolition of background rhythms. However, this is absent in 20% of cases. Brain imaging can be normal or show focal frontal atrophy. Recent studies suggest that a characteristic protein can be recovered from the spinal fluid which has high specificity but limited sensitivity for CJD.

Epidemiology

The population prevalence of CJD is approximately one per million. CJD has an incidence of 0.5 per million population per year worldwide although there may be a higher incidence in Israel. It is thought to be due to either spontaneous mutations of the human prion protein or to infection with mutated prion proteins such as occurred with a disease known as kuru that was associated with cannibalism in New Guinea. GSS is even less prevalent than CJD. Its population prevalence is unknown.

Pathology and Etiology

The predominant pathologic features of prion disease are a characteristic spongy appearance of the brain and cell loss that has given rise to the term "spongiform encephalopathy." In early onset familial cases, protein plaques are found within the spongiform degeneration.

The etiology of prion disease is thought to be an altered form of a normal brain protein known as the protease-resistant protein (PRP) or "prion" (*proteinous infectious*) protein. Prion proteins are encoded by a gene on chromosome 20 and are thought to cause the disease by acting like an infectious agent (although they do not contain DNA). Because this disease is transmissible through the transfer of the prion proteins, for many years it was thought to be due to a "slow" virus. However, no virus particle has been found and no immunologic response has been found. Several families with GSS have been described; each family carries specific mutations in the human prion protein on chromosome 20.

The pathophysiology of the disease is not known. It is presumed that prion protein becomes widely distributed in the brain and leads to neuronal injury and death with the formation of characteristic spongiform patterns. It is very likely that 100% of cases of CJD and GSS develop dementia. The presence of spongiform encephalopathy in the cortex likely explains the predominance of cortical symptoms. Ataxia and cranial nerve signs are explained by cerebellar and brain stem involvement.

4

Diseases Typically Causing Subcortical or Mixed Pattern Dementia

Chapter 4 continues a discussion begun in Chapter 3 of the most common diseases that cause dementia. In this Chapter we review diseases that typically cause a subcortical or mixed pattern of dementia. For each disease, its clinical picture, epidemiology, and pathology/etiology are discussed, in sequence.

PARKINSON DISEASE

Clinical Picture

Parkinson disease (PD) is a degenerative neurologic illness characterized by four features: a coarse "pill rolling" tremor of several beats per second usually worse at rest, rigidity or stiffness, bradykinesia or motor slowness, and poor balance.

Not all persons with PD develop dementia. In fact, until the 1980s many researchers and clinicians believed that PD did not cause dementia. While there is now universal agreement that it can, there is still debate about the criteria that should be used to diagnose dementia in PD so we prefer to use the broad definition in Table 1.1. Fewer than one-third of patients with Parkinson disease suffer from dementia at any one time. However, an additional 50% have mild cognitive impairments, most often in mental speed and flexibility. The significance of these mild cognitive changes is unknown, but their recognition is important because they may adversely affect function and well-being.

The clinical profile of the dementia of Parkinson disease is typical of

61

the subcortical dementias. The memory disorder is characterized by impaired free recall with relative preservation of recognition memory; that is, patients have difficulty spontaneously recalling information but can pick the correct response when given a right and wrong choice. Impairments in attention; verbal output (mostly with deficits in the motor aspects of speech—rate, loudness, prosody, and flow); and selection, anticipation, planning, and monitoring of goals are common. One feature atypical for subcortical dementia is impairment in visuospatial function. In the late stages of the dementia of PD, a pronounced anomia can be seen.

Patients with Parkinson disease exhibit high rates of apathy and social withdrawal that can be misinterpreted as dementia. The differentiation between apathy or slowness and dementia can be made by finding intact performance on a thorough cognitive mental status exam.

As many as 30% of patients with Parkinson disease experience visual hallucinations. Dementia is a risk factor for these hallucinations but they occur in many patients who do not have dementia. The most common hallucinations are of groups of humans or animals. Visual hallucinations are associated with the anti-Parkinson medicine levo-dopa and occur more commonly at night. Hallucinations in nonvisual modalities have also been reported in up to 12% of patients.

A major depressive syndrome develops in 30–60% of patients with PD. This prevalence is higher than reported in most other chronic neurologic disorders. The relationship between dementia and depression in PD is unclear.

Delusions, particularly paranoid or persecutory delusions, are uncommon in untreated patients but are frequent complications of pharmacotherapy. Frequencies between 3 and 8% have been reported. Dementia predisposes to delusions as do dopaminergic agents such as bromocriptine and levo-dopa.

Epidemiology

PD affects 100 per 100,000 population. This prevalence is age dependent, rising from approximately 50 per 100,000 at age 60 to approximately 130 per 100,00 at age 75. Estimates of the prevalence of dementia in Parkinson disease range from 8% to 84%, with a composite prevalence of 39%. The only prospective study found a cumulative incidence of 29%. The most significant risk factor for developing dementia is age of onset. PD beginning after age 60 is more likely to lead to dementia. Early onset Parkinson disease that is unresponsive to levo-dopa may also be a risk factor for developing dementia although this lack of response usually indicates a related disorder such as Lewy body dementia (Chapter 3) or progressive supranuclear palsy (Chapter 4).

Pathology and Etiology

Loss of dopamine-producing cells in the subcortically located substantia nigra is the basic pathologic change in Parkinson disease. Loss of 80% or more of these neurons is necessary before the clinical syndrome occurs. Degree of dopamine loss in the substantia nigra correlates with the degree of the motor disorder but its association with dementia is less clear. There is some loss of cells in the frontal lobes and the basal ganglia.

The importance of the dopamine system in this disease is further supported by the fact that the clinical syndrome responds to drugs that increase levels of brain dopamine. Treatment with dopamine agonist medications (that is, drugs that increase brain dopamine activity in some way) such as levo-dopa and bromocriptine have greatly benefitted the motor disorder. Performance on cognitive tests improves in patients treated with levo-dopa but it is not clear whether this benefit occurs in individuals with moderate or severe dementia.

Cells in the substantia nigra of Parkinson disease also contain intracellular inclusions called *Lewy bodies*. Lewy bodies may also be found in other areas of the brain, especially the nucleus basalis, the locus ceruleus, the raphe nuclei, and occasionally the cortex. Some individuals with PD dementia are found to have the pathologic findings of both AD and PD at autopsy. It is not known whether this is due to the coincident occurrence of two diseases, whether one disorder is caused by the other, or whether there is a common trigger to both. It is possible that some of the clinical variability seen in PD results from this pathologic variability.

The etiology of PD is unknown in most cases. A small percentage of cases are genetic. Toxins such as manganese and the drug MPTP cause a parkinsonian syndrome. Parkinsonism is also caused by neuroleptic medications such as haloperidol, thioridazine, risperidone, and others (see Chapter 10). Cerebrovascular disease is an uncommon etiology. The fact that PD was not described until the industrial age has led to the suggestion that environmental toxins account for many cases but this has not yet been substantiated.

PROGRESSIVE SUPRANUCLEAR PALSY

Clinical Picture

Progressive supranuclear palsy (PSP) is an uncommon disorder which resembles Parkinson disease in causing rigidity, bradykinesia (slowness), and poor balance but in which tremor does not occur. Eye movement disorder, initially presenting as a diminished or absent ability to look upward, is almost always present. The head is often thrust back due to trapezius muscle overactivity in a position referred to as "opisthotonos."

PSP was one of the first subcortical dementias to be described. Marked cognitive slowness is usually present and sometimes mimics dementia. The distinction between slowness and true dementia can be made by a careful cognitive mental status exam. For example, patients with PSP may take 10–20 seconds or longer to recall the words given in a free recall task and take 10 seconds or more for each serial seven subtraction. However, they ultimately come up with the correct answer, whereas patients with dementia do not. Some patients with PSP are *both* slow and unable to answer cognitive questions and have a subcortical form of dementia.

Visual hallucinations are common. These can be frightening and sometime cause secondary delusions, that is, delusions that arise from interpretation of the hallucinatory experience.

Epidemiology

The prevalence and incidence rates of PSP are unknown. The rate of dementia in PSP is controversial because some studies have not distinguished between slowness to respond and true inability to respond correctly.

Pathology and Etiology

Cell loss in the serotonin-producing cells of the raphe nuclei is characteristic. Other brain systems in the subcortex also degenerate. The etiology is unknown.

HUNTINGTON DISEASE

Clinical Picture

Huntington disease (HD) is an inherited, chronic, progressive condition characterized by the presence of a choreiform motor disorder and dementia. Family history follows the pattern of a dominantly inherited disease (approximately 50% of each generation is affected). A core feature of Huntington disease is the motor disorder, which has two components: (1) dyskinesias (excess movements) in the form of choreic, brief, dance-like, nonrepetitive, involuntary, and athetoid (writhing) movements of the face, limbs, and trunk, and (2) impairments of voluntary movement leading to poor coordination of fine motor skills, such as buttoning. The earliest evidence of incoordination is an eye movement disorder characterized by impaired saccade and jerky pursuit movements—that is, an inability to move the eyes smoothly when looking sideways. The motor disorders of HD cause gait instability and lead to frequent falls in the middle stages of the disease.

The clinical features of the dementia of Huntington disease are consistent with a subcortical dementia and include apathy, bradyphrenia (slowness of thinking), impaired mental flexibility, slowed thought-processing, executive dysfunction, and impaired recall. Recognition memory is relatively spared. As the disease progresses the impairments become more global, so what begins as a subcortical dementia broadens through the course of the illness to impair all cognitive capacities. The disease usually begins in midlife, although it can begin in teenage years. When it begins in the teens or early adulthood, rigidity is usually prominent early in the course of the disease.

HD is associated with high rates of depression. As many as 30% of patients suffer from depression, occasionally as the initial symptom. The depression in HD appears to run in families. Up to 10% of patients with HD develop episodes of mania in which irritability and elation are prominent. Other common noncognitive symptoms include irritability, explosiveness, and agitation. Delusions, hallucinations, and personality disturbances are less common but occur up to 10% of patients. These noncognitive symptoms can worsen the motor and cognitive impairments and may respond to symptomatic treatment with medications (see Chapter 10).

Epidemiology

HD is inherited as an autosomal dominant. The population prevalence is one per 10,000 live births. Its prevalence is similar in men and women. The average age of onset of the clinical syndrome is the late 30s to early 40s but can begin in adolescence or old age. The average patient lives 10–12 years after the development of symptoms.

Pathology and Etiology

Major strides have been made in understanding the genetics and pathophysiology of Huntington disease in recent years. It is caused by a specific mutation in a gene located on the short arm of chromosome 4. This gene contains a region in which the three amino acids cytosine (C), adenosine (A), and guanine (G) are repeated multiple times. This is called a *CAG triplet repeat*. In normal individuals, this sequence is repeated fewer than 30 times. In persons who develop HD the number of repeats is greater than 36. Earlier age of onset is associated with a higher number of repeats. Thus, individuals with 80 or more triplet repeats tend to have the earliest ages of onset, often in adolescence. Patients with greater numbers of repeats also appear to suffer from more severe disease.

The earliest pathologic change in HD is progressive shrinkage of the caudate nucleus bilaterally. In at-risk patients who carry the mutated gene, caudate atrophy can be seen on brain imaging before the clinical syndrome develops, suggesting that the brain has substantial reserve and that the clinical syndrome does not develop until a significant portion of this reserve is depleted. Several groups have reported intraneuronal, intranuclear inclusion bodies in several triplet repeat diseases including HD.

The gene product of the HD gene has been identified and is called *huntingtin*. Its function is not yet known. It appears to cause a "gain of function"—that is, the protein may cause something to occur that does not usually occur. If this is true, a preventive therapy is possible since blocking the action of this gene product might prevent brain damage from occurring.

NORMAL PRESSURE HYDROCEPHALUS

Clinical Picture

Normal pressure hydrocephalus (NPH) is a rare syndrome defined clinically by the triad of dementia, gait ataxia, and urinary incontinence. Median age of onset for NPH is in the early 70s. Prevalence is equal in men and women. It was first described in 1964 by McHugh based on autopsy findings of a normal cortical mantle, enlarged ventricles suggesting hydrocephalus, absence of an obstruction causing the hydrocephalus, and absence of specific pathology suggesting another cause.

The clinical features of the dementia reflect the periventricular subcortical locus of the pathology with impairment in executive function and memory (recall), apathy, and mental inflexibility being prominent. Rates of depression are reported to be high. Rates of mania, delusions, hallucinations, problem behaviors, and personality change are unknown.

The motor disorder of NPH is an ataxic gait disturbance with a broad-based, "magnetic" (feet seem to stick to the ground), short-stepped walk, and multistep turning. Weakness and spasticity of the legs occur late. The progression of the syndrome is fairly rapid unless treated but natural history data on large numbers of patients is not available.

Specific diagnostic criteria are not well established. The diagnosis should be suspected when the characteristic clinical triad and a subacute onset (less than 6–12 months) are present and cortical signs such as aphasia are lacking. Incontinence and apractic gait are rare early in the course of other causes of dementia. Their presence, especially in the absence of upper extremity neurologic abnormality, should raise the possibility of NPH. Imaging studies (CT, MRI) show enlarged ventricles and minimal cortical atrophy. A lumbar puncture in which withdrawal of 20 cc or more of cerebrospinal fluid (CSF) transiently improves the gait disorder supports the diagnosis. Continuous CSF pressure monitoring sometimes reveals a characteristic pattern and predicts response to shunt surgery.

Treatment is surgical and consists of placing a tube into the ventricle to drain CSF into the abdomen (peritoneum) or a central vein. The response rate to surgery is, in older studies, between 25% and 50%. With more conservative selection of subjects, response rates are higher. Within the next year, 5%–9% of patients develop serious postsurgical morbidity or die. Response can be dramatic, with complete reversal of symptoms in some cases.

Epidemiology

Based on data from referral centers, the prevalence is approximately 0.6 per 100,000 per year but the lack of a valid set of diagnostic criteria and NPH's rarity have limited epidemiologic study.

Risk factors for NPH include subarachnoid hemorrhage and meningitis. In most cases a risk factor or precipitant is not found. By definition, the risk of cognitive impairment and dementia in NPH is 100% but cases in which gait disorder and incontinence are prominent and cognitive impairment is minimal are reported. Specific criteria for the diagnosis of NPH-associated dementia are not available, so we favor the use of the dementia criteria presented in Table 1.1

Pathology and Etiology

The pathophysiology of NPH is poorly understood. Continuous monitoring of CSF pressure demonstrates an exaggeration of normal intrathecal (within the spinal fluid space) pressure waves even though CSF pressure measured on lumbar puncture is normal. These pressure waves presumably result in mechanical pressure on the subcortex surrounding the lateral and third ventricles and likely cause brain tissue destruction when the elastic properties of the brain tissue are exhausted. This may be why not all patients recover after sustained reductions in pressure.

MULTIPLE SCLEROSIS

Clinical Picture

Multiple sclerosis (MS) is a chronic neurologic disorder caused by demyelination (loss of cells surrounding nerve tracts) in the central nervous system. Its etiology is unknown. The clinical course is described as "multiple lesions in time and space." That is, diagnosis can be made with confidence when there is evidence that demyelination exists in at least two separate points in the nervous system and history suggests that these events occurred at two distinct times. MRI scanning has dramatically changed the diagnostic process since the demyelinating lesions have a distinctive character on MRI and can be found even without a corresponding clinical history or evidence on exam of neurologic abnormality. The mean age of onset is in the late 20s. Women are affected three times more than men.

The course of MS is variable. The disease is classified into three subtypes based on its clinical course. The most common subtype is the relapsing/remitting type in which neurologic impairments fluctuate over time and are intermixed with periods of months or years in which the patient's condition is stable. This type affects as many as half of MS patients. Approximately one-third of patients are affected by the secondarily progressive form of MS, which begins as the relapsing/remitting type but develops into a steady neurologic decline. The third subtype is progressive from its very onset. This form has the worst prognosis and highest likelihood of developing dementia.

Given that MS is a demyelinating disease and myelinated tracts are subcortical in locations, it is not surprising that the MS-associated dementia follows a subcortical pattern with impairments in information processing, memory retrieval, executive function, and disregulation of mood.

Clinical series suggest that 16%–20% of MS patients have mood disorders, the majority suffering from major depression. A smaller number (4%–5%) suffers panic disorder. Sustained euphoria, irritability, and hypomanic syndromes occur but are infrequent. Delusions and hallucinations are rare.

An emotional state characterized by lack of concern is associated with the dementia of MS. Called "eutonia" by the British neurologist Kinnier-Wilson and often referred to as "euphoria," this mood state is uncommon but associated with poor adaptation, probably because it is associated with a lack of awareness of the extent of impairment.

Epidemiology

The population prevalence of MS is 170 per 100,000. In community settings, 4% of MS patients suffer from dementia. This number rises to 8%–10% in clinical settings. As many as 20% additional patients with MS have measurable but mild cognitive impairments but their significance and impact on functioning are relatively small.

The main risk factor for dementia in MS is involvement of specific white matter areas in the brain: the corona radiata, the insula, and the hippocampus. No other clear risk factors for dementia in MS have been identified. Criteria for dementia in MS have not been published.

Pathology and Etiology

The pathophysiology of MS is thought to be autoimmune damage of the myelin sheath of nerve tracts, perhaps triggered by a viral illness that occurred earlier in life. Not surprisingly, the location of white matter lesions is crucial to the development of dementia symptoms. The scattered nature of the subcortical lesions explains the variable clinical picture. For example, patients present with executive dysfunction or unconcern if frontal/anterior white matter areas are affected, but memory disorders if lateral temporal areas are involved.

HIV INFECTION AND AIDS

Clinical Picture

Cognitive impairments have been associated with HIV infection since AIDS was first identified in 1981. AIDS-associated dementia can be divided into two types. Opportunistic brain infection or lymphoma causes a mixture of cortical and subcortical symptoms depending on the site of injury. For example, brain toxoplasmosis usually causes a subcortical pattern of dementia while brain cryptococcosis is usually associated with a mixed pattern of language disturbance, affective change, and executive dysfunction.

The second type of AIDS-associated dementia is caused by the HIV virus itself. It is a subcortical dementia with memory loss, slowed mental processing, and executive dysfunction. It usually develops in an insidious and progressive fashion. Reduced motor speed and impaired nonverbal memory are prominent. In early stages the most serious impairments are in tests of planning which are detected on the Grooved Pegboard or the Trail Making Test.

The most common noncognitive symptoms of HIV dementia are personality change, apathy, social withdrawal, and disinterest. HIV dementia is associated with the development of manic syndromes in patients with no genetic or personal risk for mood disorders. In the 12–18 months before AIDS, 10%–15% of patients develop a new episode of depression.

HIV dementia is associated with a motor disorder characterized by poor coordination, slowness of movement, extrapyramidal symptoms, postural instability, and falling. Prior to the development of multiple drug therapy, AIDS-dementia had a poor prognosis. With retroviral therapy the cognitive decline can be slowed. Without treatment, AIDS-dementia portends a poor prognosis and rapid decline: Typical survival is 6 months or less.

The main risk factors for HIV-associated dementia are low hemoglobin, low body mass index, high prevalence of constitutional symptoms, and older age at onset. Reductions in pre-AIDS hemoglobin are the most significant predictor. Cognitive impairment becomes much more prevalent after the CD4 cell counts drop below 100.

Epidemiology

The prevalence of HIV infection varies throughout the world; western industrialized countries and South American countries are least affected. The most rapid increases in prevalence are in Africa and Asia, especially Southeast Asia. The World Health Organization estimates that as many as 30 million worldwide will be infected by the virus by the time the pandemic has reached its peak. In the United States it is estimated that about 750,000 people are infected with the HIV virus. Well over 500,000 cases of AIDS have been reported in the United States, more than half in the last few years. There has been a decline in new AIDS cases in the United States since 1995 when new powerful antiviral therapies were introduced.

Up to 60% of AIDS patients experience cognitive difficulty prior to death but a prominent dementia syndrome is present in approximately 15%. The incidence of dementia in HIV infected patients is 7% per year.

Cognitive impairment has been reported in the early stages of HIV infection when the CD4 cell count is greater than 500. However, longitudinal studies have found that these cognitive impairments are not progressive. This suggests that these impairments existed prior to the HIV disease.

Pathology and Etiology

The HIV virus initiates and sustains the dementia through direct infection of brain macrophages or microglia cells that normally fight infection in the brain. Neurons and other brain cells, such as glial astrocytes, are not directly infected. Thus, brain injury and dementia are not the direct result of virus-induced neuronal death. Rather, two "indirect" neurotoxic processes are involved. In one, the virus induces the expression of viral proteins on the surface of macrophages that are toxic to neurons. A second and more destructive mechanism is immune dysregulation in the brain. The infected microglia produce several cytokines or proteins that are directly neurotoxic. How or why this action becomes localized in the subcortex is not known.

The HIV virus enters the central nervous system early in the course of infection. Opportunistic infections are commonly associated with the later stages of HIV disease and include toxoplasmosis, cryptococcosis, tuberculosis, and syphilis. Additionally, there is an increase in brain lymphomas that can cause cognitive impairment. At autopsy as many as 80% of patients have pathologic markers indicating HIV infection in the brain.

DEMENTIA ASSOCIATED WITH MOOD DISORDERS

Clinical Picture

The mood disorders are characterized by abnormalities in mood, self-attitude, and vital sense or physical well-being. Depressed individuals of all ages complain of cognitive difficulty but measurable cognitive impairment is seen primarily in the elderly. We will refer to this form of mood-associated thinking impairment as *depression-induced cognitive impairment* ("DICI") since not all patients fulfill criteria for dementia.

The clinical picture of DICI approximates the phenomenology of a subcortical dementia. Patients with depressive dementia have impairments in free recall, delayed recall, and verbal delayed memory but typically have intact delayed visual memory and intact recognition memory. Some depressed patients have decreased verbal fluency, slowed responses, and difficulty with naming.

A reversible motor disorder consisting of bradykinesia and stooped posture has been described in some patients with depression. This, too, occurs predominantly in the elderly. Since these features simulate the syndrome of Parkinson disease, this motor disorder may be due to impairments in basal ganglia function. Mania is accompanied by impaired cognitive performance but there is so little study of this condition that we will not discuss it further.

Depression is also associated with many irreversible dementias including Alzheimer disease, vascular dementia, Parkinson disease, and Huntington disease and is probably induced by the neuropathology of these diseases. It is sometimes the first or presenting symptom of these conditions. The pattern of the dementia reflects the anatomic location of the underlying disease.

The concept of *pseudo-dementia*—that is, depression imitating dementia—has been replaced by the recognition that the co-occurrence of depression and dementia often presages a progressive dementia but can indicate a reversible dementia due to major depression. Criteria to distinguish these are yet to be validated by long term follow-up studies. The hypothesis that there are two broad syndromes of depression-associated cognitive impairment has been confirmed in one postmortem study in which 42% of a small sample of patients with "affective psychosis" had neuritic plaques and neurofibrillary tangles consistent with Alzheimer disease while the remainder had normal neuropathology.

Depression is associated with increased mortality but no studies have determined whether depression increases the mortality rate associated with dementia.

Epidemiology

The incidence and prevalence of dementia associated with mood disorder are a matter of considerable debate. Among hospitalized patients whose onset of depression is late in life, 30%–40% evidence symptoms of DICI during the depression. Prevalence is much lower in outpatients.

Pathology and Etiology

The etiology of dementia in depression is not well understood. CT and MRI studies find more cortical atrophy in patients with major depression than elderly controls and some studies find a greater number of white matter hyperintensities in depressed individuals. These changes are most marked in patients whose depression has begun in late life. Thus, the development of cognitive impairment in a patient with depression can be explained in three ways. Major depression with onset in later life can be the first symptom of a degenerative or vascular dementia. Second, depression and dementia may have the same cause but both manifestations may not always be present. Alexopoulos has suggested the term "vascular depression" be applied to late onset cases with evidence of brain vascular disease. Presumably, this pathology also contributes to the development of cognitive impairment. Finally, aging may diminish the brain's reserve and this could be further "unmasked" by depression. That is, depression might place a physiologic burden on the brain systems that underlie cognition and induce impaired performance only when the depression is present. We believe each of these mechanisms is at work and that more than one may contribute in a single patient.

CEREBROVASCULAR DISEASE

Clinical Picture

Strokes due to cerebrovascular disease are the second leading cause of death in the United States and cerebrovascular disease is the second most common cause of dementia. In the past, this type of dementia was referred to as *multi-infarct dementia* or *stroke-related dementia*. At present the term *vascular dementia* is preferred because aspects of brain vascular disease besides stroke (for example, hypoxia) may be responsible for cognitive impairment. Table 4.1 contains the National Institute for Neurologic Disorders and Stroke-Association International pour la Recherdie et l'Enseignement en Neurosciences (NINDS-AIRENS) diagnostic criteria for vascular dementia.

Vascular dementia presents in two broad clinical subtypes. The first is related to multiple small and/or large thromboembolic brain infarcts. The characteristics of the clinical syndrome depend on the location of the infarcts and thus may have mixed cortical and subcortical features. Common symptoms include amnesia, receptive or expressive aphasia, constructional or other types of apraxia, and dysfunctions associated with injury of the frontal lobes, including executive disturbance. These impairments reflect the anatomy of the cerebral vasculature and the frequent occurrence of strokes in the temporal, parietal and frontal cortical regions.

The second subtype of vascular dementia results from the degeneration of subcortical white matter, referred to as leukoareosis, and is presumed due to long standing vascular insufficiency in deep brain areas. Memory disturbance, executive dysfunction, apathy, and amotivation are prominent. Brain imaging and gross pathologic studies show extensive white matter loss (leukoareosis). The extreme degree of this condition is known as Binswanger disease and is associated with chronic, poorly controlled hypertension.

Multi-infarct dementia has been said to progress in a step-wise pattern. However, many pathologically documented cases of multi-infarct/

Table 4.1. Criteria for Vascular Disease Causing Dementia

A. Dementia
   Decline by examination and objective testing
   Deficits in memory PLUS two other areas of cognition
   Functional impairment

B. Cerebrovascular Disease by History, Examination, or Imaging

C. A Relationship Between *A* and *B*
   Dementia onset within 3 months of Cerebrovascular Accident
   Cognitive change is stepwise, abrupt, or fluctuating
   Strokes affect critical areas

D. Supportive features
   Early presence of gait disturbance
   Early presence of urinary frequency or incontinence
   Typical neurologic examination findings

E. Consciousness Intact

vascular dementia have followed a slowly progressive course. An insidiously progressive course is more common in the leukoareotic type of vascular dementia. Patients with vascular dementia tend to die sooner and become debilitated more rapidly than patients with Alzheimer disease.

Vascular dementia is associated with several noncognitive impairments. A depressive syndrome affects 50%–60% of patients. A variety of personality changes can be seen. In the disinhibited type, socially inappropriate behaviors or intermittent but frequent mood swings occur with minimal or no provocation. Stimulus bound behavior—that is, an inability to stop responding to a stimulus (for example, grabbing food whenever it is seen or urinating in trash cans)—is a common associated problem. Apathy, profound slowness, disinterest, and resistance to care can also be seen or associated with vascular dementia. Delusions and hallucinations are also common in vascular dementia, especially in association with strokes of the nondominant hemisphere. Associated neurologic features, such as paresis (weakness), paralysis, cranial nerve changes, visual field loss, sensory defects, or seizures occur depending on the location of the stroke.

Epidemiology

The risk of dementia after a clinically evident stroke is not fully known. One study suggests that after 3 months as many as 13% of new stroke patients suffer from dementia. Another study provides an estimate closer to 10% after 6 months. Four years after a stroke as many as 33% of patients develop dementia. Autopsy series of patients with the old definition of multi-infarct indicate that 30%–50% have the pathology of both cerebrovascular accidents and of Alzheimer disease. Vascular dementia has a median age of onset in the early 70s and may decrease in incidence thereafter. It affects men more than women.

The primary risk factors for stroke—hypertension, hypercholesterolemia, and diabetes—increase the likelihood that dementia will develop after a stroke, probably because a greater number of strokes increases the likelihood that dementia will develop. Controlling these risk factors reduces the incidence and progression of vascular dementia.

Pathology and Etiology

Vascular dementia follows the "mass action" principle: The greater the amount of brain tissue affected, the greater the likelihood and severity of dementia. Dementia is likely when 50 cc of brain tissue is infarcted. The pattern of symptoms depends primarily on the location of injury.

There are several mechanisms of stroke and each causes a different form of dementia. In *embolic strokes*, atherosclerotic plaque breaks off from larger arteries (most often the carotid arteries in the neck) or the heart, travels to the brain, and blocks the blood vessels at the point at which the diameter of the plaque exceeds the diameter of the artery. This causes sudden death of tissue downstream from the blockage because cells are deprived of blood and oxygen. *Thrombotic strokes* are due to the formation of a clot in the artery, usually in association with an arteriosclerotic plaque. The clot closes off blood flow downstream, leading to tissue death. Both embolic and thrombotic stroke come on suddenly. In *hypertensive vasculopathy,* smaller penetrating arteries of the subcortex become narrowed from long standing high blood pressure. This leads to oxygen and nutrient starvation and probably demyelination. The clinical picture is usually of a slowly progressive subcortical dementia without localizing neurologic signs. Another stroke mechanism is rupture of arteries or aneurysm which leads to hemorrhagic (bleeding) stroke. This can result in massive deficits because of loss of blood flow and the mechanical effects of bleeding into a close space. Stroke can also occur if there is a sudden drop in systemic blood pressure, such as during a heart attack or cardiac arrest, or loss of nutrient supply induced by hypoglycemia or hypoxia.

TRAUMATIC BRAIN INJURY

Clinical Picture

The clinical features of dementia after traumatic brain injury (TBI) vary by the site of the injury. Cortical, subcortical, and mixed patterns of impairment may occur. In closed head injury, the most common feature is amnesia, with difficulty learning new material. Frontal lobe dysfunctions are frequent as well. Loss of highly learned motor skills, executive dysfunction, language disturbance, inattention, poor concentration, and apraxia can occur. After a penetrating head injury the impairments are often more focal and relate to the areas where penetration occurred.

Personality change and mood disturbance are the most common behavioral disorders after TBI, occurring in 50%–75% of cases of moderate to severe head injury. Symptoms include disinhibition, apathy, loss of motivation, depression, explosiveness, trouble concentrating, and memory loss.

The *postconcussion syndrome* consists of headache, fatigue, and inattention. It is a common sequela of mild head injury. Depressive syndromes and mania also occur after head injury in the absence of dementia and can worsen cognitive performance. Depression afflicts as many as 25%–30% of patients in the first year following the TBI and mania affects up to 5% of patients. Most studies suggest that the mood and cognitive syndromes are independent. Delusions and hallucinations are uncommon. Neurologic impairment after TBI relates to region of injury.

Epidemiology

More than 500,000 cases of head trauma occur yearly in the United States. Perhaps a third to half of all traumatic brain injuries are moderate to severe in nature. While as many as 40% of patients develop transient or permanent amnesia after moderate or severe head injury, a smaller number, about 8%–10%, develop a dementia syndrome.

Specific risk factors for dementia after traumatic brain injury have not been identified, but it is likely that indicators of poor outcome after traumatic brain injury increase the risk for dementia. These include low initial score on the Glasgow Coma Scale (a measure of injury severity that grades the clinical status of the patient at the time of the original injury), older patient age, high velocity closed head injury, injury to other body areas, brain lesions before the injury, increased intracranial pressure at the time of the injury, longer duration of coma, longer in-hospital stay after the injury, and poor premorbid cognitive state. The criteria for dementia in Table 1.1 are best used.

Pathology and Etiology

A variety of mechanisms contribute to trauma of the brain after a blow to the head. Penetrating injuries, in which objects such as bullets or spokes enter through the skull, cause a focal or tract-type mechanical injury. Rapid acceleration and deceleration of the head cause movement of the brain within the skull, which leads to two types of injury. Mechanical injury to brain areas next to the skull is caused when the relatively plastic brain strikes the immovable skull. This damage tends to be most severe in the orbitofrontal area because the brain rubs against the floor of the skull in the front and in the inferior temporal areas where the brain can hit against the petrous bones. Acceleration and deceleration can also cause stretching of the axons of the descending and ascending tracts.

Mechanical trauma and axonal shearing also cause hemorrhage, inflammation, edema, and mass effects and these combine to cause damage or death to brain structures. Further injury can result from epidural, subdural, and intracerebral hematomas. The principal determinant of damage is the amount of energy imparted to the brain, the amount of brain tissue directly injured either through *coup* (the site of the blow) or *countercoup* (the brain hitting the opposite side of the skull) injury, and the location of the injury. Global cognitive syndromes such as inattention, headache, and difficulty concentrating may be the result of "mass action," that is, a diffuse disruption of brain cell function, but it is more likely that the specific features of dementia in any individual are closely related to the location of the most severely affected areas of the brain. For example, after coup/countercoup acceleration and deceleration injuries, memory disturbance results from injury to the temporal lobe; executive dysfunction from frontal trauma; and inattention/poor concentration from damage to the reticular activating and related systems.

TOXIC DEMENTIAS

Several substances have been associated with central nervous system toxicity. Alcohol is the most widely used such substance. Other substances with a propensity for inducing abuse and dependence that may cause cognitive impairments with chronic use include cocaine, opiates, marijuana, sedative-hypnotics, and solvent inhalants (benzene, glue, toluene, turpentine). Heavy metals such as lead, arsenic, mercury, manganese, and thallium are also injurious to the brain.

Clinical Picture

The clinical syndrome of alcohol-related dementia is varied. A mixture of cortical and subcortical features has been described; the most prominent impairments occur in memory. Recall and recognition are equally disturbed, and there is executive dysfunction. However, the inhalant substances, such as glue and toluene, may cause executive dysfunctions predominantly Early recognition is important since some or all of the deficits can reverse with abstinence and good nutrition.

Epidemiology

A discussion of the epidemiology of alcohol use and of other substances of abuse is beyond the scope of this chapter. Alcoholism afflicts 15%–20% of the U.S. population and the combined prevalence of other substances of abuse, excluding nicotine and caffeine, is approximately 5%. The epidemiology of heavy metal intoxication in adults is much less well known but occupational exposure is a clear risk factor. In children, exposure to lead remains a major public health problem. As many as 10% of those who develop alcohol use disorders develop dementia. Dementia related to alcoholism accounts for less than 2% of all dementias, however.

Risk factors for developing dementia in the context of chronic alcoholism are not well understood. Duration and amount of alcohol are major risk factors and a family history of alcoholism may be contributory. Alcohol abuse predisposes to repeated head trauma and nutritional deprivation, both of which can cause dementia. The epidemiology of cognitive disorders in persons with polysubstance and inhalant abuse and with heavy metal and solvent exposure is not well established

Pathology and Etiology

The pathophysiology of dementia syndromes due to toxins is poorly understood. It is not clear if alcohol itself is the cause of the dementia or whether the nutritional disorders and head trauma associated with alcohol abuse are the primary culprits. All probably contribute variably in different individuals. Autopsies of persons with alcoholism and dementia reveal damage to the mammillary bodies, the dorsomedial nucleus of the thalamus, the nucleus basalis, the hippocampus, the amygdala, and the cerebellum. The association between these pathologic findings and the dementia syndrome is suggestive but not definitive. The brain atrophy on CT and MRI scans seen in patients with alcohol abuse can be reversed with abstinence. Wernicke-Korsakoff syndrome is characterized by amnesia, gait disturbance, and impaired eye movements and is due to a thiamine deficiency that damages the dorsomedial nucleus of the thalamus or the mammillary bodies. It is likely caused by malnutrition secondary to alcoholism and occurs in genetically vulnerable individuals.

Little is known about the neuropathologic and neurophysiologic changes that contribute to the development of dementia caused by the use and exposure to other toxic substances. It is plausible that inhalants enter the brain through the cribriform plate at the base of the frontal lobes and cause executive dysfunction by a direct toxic mechanism, but this has not been proven.

Overview of
Dementia Care

The care of patients with dementia is based on six general principles (Table 5.1). Each of these rests on the belief that knowledge of the patient's wishes and goals prior to the illness should guide care. This is easy in the abstract but can be difficult when problems are persistent or severe. It is also easy to lose sight of the fact that small changes can be of great value.

GOALS OF CARE

The goals of treatment are determined by the needs of the individual patient and his or her caregivers. Table 5.2 lists the most common needs of patients and families. The goals that follow from them are discussed below. An accurate diagnosis is usually the first goal. This is met by determining that dementia is present, classifying it, and identifying its cause (Chapters 2, 3, and 4). When new problems develop, whether cognitive, medical, psychological, behavioral, or functional, accurate reassessment and diagnosis of the new problems becomes a priority.

The next goal of treatment is to treat and, if possible, cure the disease which has caused the dementia. Unfortunately, cure is rarely possible at present.

A third goal of dementia care is symptom relief. Reaching this goal requires an understanding of the specific symptoms of each patient and creativity in devising treatment approaches. Three types of symptoms are evident in most dementia patients: cognitive, functional, and behav-

Table 5.1. Six Principles of Dementia Care

1. People with dementia are individuals
2. People with dementia have the same human needs as others
3. People with dementia have the same human value as other adults
4. People with dementia can be healthy and happy
5. Small changes can have great practical value
6. Something can always be done to help

ioral. Each should be addressed, sometimes separately, but sometimes with a single approach. In Alzheimer disease, cognitive symptoms can be improved in the short term by medications (Chapter 10). Behavioral symptoms and declines in functioning can be treated in many dementias. These are discussed in Chapters 8 and 9.

The provision of appropriate supportive care to the patient is a fourth goal (Chapter 6). This includes ensuring meaningful activity and personal safety and addressing physical and dental health needs. Good supportive care requires knowledgeable caregivers and a supportive, stable environment.

A final goal of care is the support of the family and other caregivers (Chapter 7). It is achieved by educating about the diagnosis and prognosis of the patient's condition, providing guidance in decision-making, helping families adjust to the changes brought about in their own lives,

Table 5.2. Needs of Dementia Patients and Their Families

Patients Need	Families Need
Accurate diagnosis	Education about diagnosis
Treatment of the disease	Prognosis
Treatment of cognitive symptoms	Guidance in decision-making
Treatment of behavioral symptoms	Emotional support
Support of declines in functioning	Referral to community resources
Provision for needs and wants	Physical and emotional well-being
Meaningful activity	Socialization
Personal safety	Time for themselves
Adequate physical health	
A supportive stable environment	

and referring to community resources. Family members also need to attend to their own physical, emotional, and social well being.

TREATMENT PLANNING

The treatment plan provides a blueprint for care. The attributes of an optimal dementia treatment plan are that it must be (1) Realistic, (2) Flexible, (3) Anticipatory, (4) Comprehensive, (5) Hopeful. A plan must be rational and realistic; recommendations should be based on a thorough assessment of each patient and caregiver at every point in time. Although much is known about the course of dementia, there is variability among patients. The use of interventions should be based on a realistic sense of their likelihood for success. False hope can be as destructive as no hope. The optimal treatment plan should be dynamic and flexible—it must change if the patient's or caregiver's condition changes. If a crisis occurs, ready access to the appropriate professional is crucial. Since much of day-to-day care rests on trial and error, the plan must be flexible enough to address the unexpected.

An effective treatment plan should be anticipatory. Preventing a problem before it develops is ideal, although not always possible. For example, providing a medical alert bracelet and keeping recent photographs available in case a patient wanders away can save a life. The plan should prepare for most eventualities that are common to dementia. For example, informing family members that swallowing problems are just beginning to develop will allow them to consider the benefits and burdens of tube feeding well before they are faced with the need to make a decision. Teaching family members that behavioral symptoms can be due to the dementing disease might encourage them to seek help for distressing mental symptoms and prevent them from taking personally something said by the patient as the result of a delusion or memory impairment.

The optimal treatment plan should also be comprehensive and focus on as many aspects of the patient's care and caregivers' needs as possible. Since caregivers carry out the treatment plan, communication between them and the clinician is a necessity. It is sometimes best if there is a spokesperson for the family, but the key to success is continued communication among the interested parties.

A comprehensive dementia plan should include day-to-day activities for the patient, indicate which signs and symptoms should be brought to the attention of a professional, provide a list of which professionals are involved in their care and what aspects of care they are addressing, and specify the plan for future transitions, such as nursing home placement.

A critical element of the treatment plan is the conveyance of hopefulness. The plan should assume that short term improvement is possible, but recognize that, in most cases, long-term decline is inevitable. As is true in the care of any chronic illness, the focus is on maximizing functions and minimizing disability by identifying those impairments that can be treated.

IMPLEMENTING THE TREATMENT PLAN

The implementation of the treatment plan begins with the communication of the diagnosis and treatment options to the patient and family. The most effective way to communicate diagnosis is in a family conference. This involves inviting into the office or clinic all members of the family who will potentially be involved in caring for the patient.

The discussion of diagnosis and treatment options should be as clear and concise as possible. There should be time to answer questions and an opportunity for all involved to raise concerns. By meeting together, all family members hear about the specific difficulties the patient is experiencing and how they are a product of disease. It is sometimes the case that family members who are not providing direct care do not appreciate how arduous caregiving is. The clinician should listen for this and clarify misunderstandings on this issue. We usually meet without the patient first since many family members do not ask questions if the patient is present and because the patient usually becomes "talked about" rather than being included. We then have the patient join the meeting and review the treatment options, allowing the patient to set the pace of discussion.

Many family members benefit from written instructions and information. Useful guidelines and information pamphlets about dementia are available through the Alzheimer's and Related Disorders Association in the United States and similar information is available in other countries from comparable societies.

Several questions are frequently asked. One is, "How was the diagnosis established?" Clinicians need to explain the process of diagnosis, as presented in Chapter 2, emphasizing its systematic and time-tested nature. A review of the results of cognitive testing, such as specific items or scores on the cognitive MMSE and neuropsychological testing, is sometimes useful since they objectively identify deficits. Patients and families sometimes explain deficits on single items, e.g., trouble with knowing the date or doing the serial sevens, by saying the patient was anxious or "never could do this," or using statements such as "No old person can do this." We find it helpful to remind families that it is important to look at the big picture ("Yes, one or two problems on the examination might be due to anxiety but not ten items"), that these tests are generally well normed by age ("Most older people score above 25 on MMSE"), that declines are more relevant than absolute scores ("Your husband was a college graduate who likely would have scored 28–30 on the MMSE years ago, so a score of 22 today is a decline"), and that all patients tested in the clinic are anxious but that anxiety rarely accounts for consistently poor performance.

Other frequently asked questions at the time of diagnosis include, "How sure are you of this?" "What can be done?" and "What does this mean for the future?" Patients and families should be reminded that the diagnosis of dementia is based on the presence of a clinical syndrome and can be made with very high confidence while the accuracy of a diagnosis of the specific cause of dementia varies, ranging from around 100% for posttraumatic dementias, to 90% for Alzheimer disease, to as low as 50%–60% for vascular dementia without Alzheimer disease. When discussing what can be done, the clinician should review the treatment recommendations, options, and expected outcomes of each.

Providing information about the future course of the disease (prognosis) is more difficult. We believe that clinicians should provide an estimate of progression if they have an opinion but be very clear about the limited ability of any clinician to predict the future. The accuracy of the prognostic assessment becomes more accurate as patients are followed over time and the course of that individual becomes evident. The rate of worsening in dementia is intimately tied to its cause. Alzheimer disease patients decline on average 4 points on the MMSE every year. Vascular dementia may not decline at all, even though the decline is more rapid than Alzheimer disease on average. The rate of decline in AIDS-dementia has slowed since the development of antiviral therapies.

Involving the patient with dementia in the treatment planning process is important. This begins with establishing a relationship with the patient (see Chapter 6). However, many patients with dementia, particularly those with Alzheimer, lack insight into their cognitive deficits. This lack of insight is called an *nosoagnosia*. Persistent attempts to convince patients without insight that they suffer from dementia are rarely useful and often may lead to distress. Confrontation almost never helps. Some patients have an awareness that something is wrong and complain that "I'm not right and need to be put back together" or "There is something different about me" but deny having a memory problem. We recommend telling them once that they have a memory problem, but if they deny it, then going on to tell them that you will do your best to solve their problem. If the patient has a different complaint, it should be responded to as well as possible. However, if patients accept that something is wrong because their spouse says so, it is usually not necessary to persuade them that they have dementia.

Communication among caregivers is obviously important. Caregivers vary in their time availability, devotion, energy, and resources. The clinician's primary responsibility is for the well being of the patient, although the well being of caregiver and patient is inextricably intertwined. We try to be direct with caregivers and to communicate freely. We are not always successful but believe that the themes of this book—being informed about dementia, focusing on problem solving, acknowledging and addressing the emotional impact of dementia, and reexamining the patient's condition when problems arise—are keys to good communication.

Caring for dementia patients often requires a multidisciplinary team. The team may include primary care physicians, medical specialists (psychiatrists, neuropsychiatrists, neurologists, geriatricians), psychologists, nurses, social workers, counselors, activity therapists, occupational therapists, and physical therapists. It is important that all professionals involved in treatment participate in the development of a plan. Regular communication between team members is necessary. At times of crisis, for example, when a patient is hospitalized, it is useful to have a face-to-face meeting of the treatment team.

Every member of the treatment team has unique skills. The need for several care-providers has led to the suggestion that a care coordinator be appointed for each patient to coordinate the professionals. In practice, the family or a family spokesperson, in collaboration with a physician or nurse, becomes the care coordinator for most patients.

Clinicians should strive to include rather than exclude practitioners from different backgrounds and to see all different practitioners as colleagues. It is often a relief for professionals to be reassured that they are not expected to know, understand, or do everything. Sometimes the family must be reminded or encouraged to use practitioners who have specific backgrounds. They may need legal, financial, medical, social, or transportation resources. Social workers are an important source of knowledge about the community since they may know who can provide information about specific problems. If there is a local Alzheimer's Association chapter or similar organization, it too might provide information about specific agencies that may be able to help. In most cases, the medical care of patients with dementia can be managed in the community by a primary care physician in collaboration with other professionals. Occasionally, specialists need to be consulted.

The treatment plan's implementation should address the setting in which the patient is treated. Care is provided in settings as diverse as outpatient medical clinics, supported housing (assisted living, residential care, life care, group homes), adult day care, hospital wards, psychiatric inpatient units, or nursing homes. It is important to consider how the patient's needs are being met by each site and to understand how the strengths and weaknesses of the setting interact with the patient's needs (see discussion later in this chapter).

Care providers should try to anticipate the issues that may arise when moving to a different care setting. Transitions in housing (see Chapter 6) are particularly challenging and are often associated with increased confusion and behavioral disturbance. These usually remit as patients become familiar with the new setting. A frequent question about moving is whether it is better to move a person earlier or later in the course of the illness. This question is best addressed on an individual basis but often there is no single right answer.

GOOD CLINICAL PRACTICES

Table 5.3 presents a list of good clinical practices professionals should keep in mind when they care for dementia patients. This book provides some basic facts about the most common diseases causing dementia, but further reading may be necessary in complicated cases. An appreciation of the natural history assists the clinician in determining whether a problem is related to disease progression or if an alternative cause should be sought. For example, if a patient with Alzheimer disease declines more rapidly than is expected, the clinician should look for a cause—such as depression or a urinary tract infection—to explain the decline.

Knowledge of the current status of each specific patient requires an adequate diagnostic evaluation and formulation as well as regular up-

Table 5.3. Good Clinical Practices in Dementia Care

Know the natural history of the disease
Know the specific case
Know the available local resources
Use a team approach
Use persistent trial-and-error problem solving
Think of how to deal with a crisis before it happens
Be as specific as possible
Be aware of sudden change

dates about how the patient is doing, who the involved caregivers are, and which other professionals have been consulted. Careful record keeping in the patient's chart helps keep the care team abreast of changes in a person's condition. We recommend a routine visit approximately every 6 months. This is an optimal interval for following the progression of the disease and keeping the clinician aware of the person's current status.

Good practice also includes knowing the available local resources. This is easier for those who specialize in dementia care, but most practitioners come into contact with relatively few patients with dementia. Knowing who to refer to can substitute for knowing specific resources. Resources include names of social workers or rehabilitation experts (occupational/physical therapists) who specialize in dementia; local specialty or university clinics specializing in dementia; and specific service programs such as adult daycare programs, senior centers, supported living environments, and nursing homes that specialize in patients with dementia.

Trial-and-error problem solving is a crucial element of dementia care. Even the most experienced clinician is confronted with situations that seem daunting. No obvious solution may be at hand or the problem may require time to solve. Almost always, something can be done to improve a situation. Therefore, the clinician should be ready to try several things, to be persistent, to recognize failure when it occurs, and to try new alternatives when failure does occur.

An important aspect of good clinical practice is to identify changes in the patient's state and to teach caregivers how to do this. Many changes are an inevitable part of dementia progression. Others are not. A sudden change should alert the family and caregiver to the likelihood that a new problem has occurred. In the patient with Alzheimer disease, the development of a new problem should raise questions about a new medical condition, medication toxicity, or a new brain lesion such as a stroke. Any sudden change should be considered treatable until proven otherwise. When a significant change occurs, it is good practice to review in detail all changes that occurred in the patient's environment over the past month or 6 weeks. The addition of a new medicine, changes in the routine of a daycare program, a new caregiver, illness in a caregiver, or an unwitnessed fall can all cause the patient to change.

Clinicians who care for patients with dementia should be prepared to deal with crises. Crises in dementia care seem to occur at the most inopportune moments and often inconvenience everyone. When they occur, the first step is to get as much information as possible as quickly as possible. How much of the crisis relates to the patient, how much relates to the care-provider, and how much relates to the environment should be determined. The next step is to engage the caregiver in a conversation (often on the phone) to help them calm down and to problem solve. This conversation should review what the caregiver has tried and note what has and what has not helped. Determining the availability of other caregivers may be important. Even though caregivers don't always do what is advised, talking to a professional on the phone can help deescalate the situation, introduce logic to the situation, and offer possible solutions.

Medical emergencies must be attended to. It may be necessary to have the patient evaluated at an emergency room or hospitalized, particularly if there is evidence that something dangerous is about to happen. Emergency department visits should be viewed as a last resort because ERs are not well equipped to handle patients with dementia and will often restrain them due to lack of staffing or inexperience.

DEMENTIA IN SPECIAL POPULATIONS

The symptoms of dementia depend on the disease causing it but are modified by the characteristics of each individual. A knowledge of features common to many individuals forms the basis for effective care, but some groups of patients are different enough to require special discussion.

Dementia in the Young

Dementia is uncommon before age 65. It is extremely rare in early adulthood because most of the diseases that cause dementia in the young are rare genetic conditions. One major difference between dementia in the young and in the elderly is the effect on the family. If the patient has young children, the disease often has a devastating effect on their lives. Marital relationships are more likely to be disrupted, perhaps because the couple may not have developed sufficient bonding to survive the devastation of the illness. Since younger patients are more likely to be working, change in work performance is sometimes the first symptom. Loss of a job may occur before the dementia is recognized as the cause for declining ability, depriving them of disability income. Even with disability insurance, they will have had less time to accumulate savings, so financial problems are much more common in young patients.

Cultural and Ethnic Background

Few studies have looked at how cultural and ethnic background affect the clinical presentation of dementia, but anecdotal writings and clinical experience suggest a wide variation. In some cultural groups, dementia is not seen as an illness but as an aspect of growing old. In others, it is seen as the result of lifestyle. It is important for the clinician to recognize how memory loss and cognitive decline are viewed in persons of different cultural and ethnic backgrounds and to use this knowledge in devising a care plan.

Cultural and economic status also influence the availability of and willingness to use resources. If there is mistrust of traditional medicine, individuals may be reluctant to use desired or necessary services. The appropriateness of support groups also varies significantly by culture. While it is sometimes said that support groups are a uniquely American phenomenon, there are many cultural groups in the United States for whom speaking in public about ill family members is not acceptable, especially if strangers are present. Other supports will probably benefit such families more.

The Adult with Mental Retardation

Individuals with lifelong cognitive incapacities such as mental retardation are at greater risk for dementia. In Down syndrome, for example, the onset of Alzheimer disease is common in midlife. Variations in the initial presentation and course of dementia are among the challenges of identifying and treating dementia in the mentally retarded. Early changes in behavior are sometimes wrongly attributed to changing life circumstances when they are the result of the onset of Alzheimer disease. Conversely, changes in behavior due to depression or a reaction to change in life circumstances may be misinterpreted as due to dementia.

DEMENTIA IN SPECIFIC ENVIRONMENTS

Day Programs

Many day programs have been developed to provide activities, supportive care, and supervision to impaired older persons. A substantial portion of persons in adult day care suffer from dementia. One controversy is whether it is better to keep healthy elders and persons with dementia in separate programs. Our experience suggests that combined programming is not appropriate and often not beneficial to the cognitively normal older person. The hope that the mingling of persons with dementia and normal cognition would provide for a better understanding of dementia and provide stimulation for the person with dementia is far outweighed by the need of individuals with dementia for more direction and cognitive support. While some literature suggests that integration of cognitively intact and impaired individuals results in increased depression in those cognitively intact, we know of no studies which support this or the opposing position.

Another controversial issue is whether there should be a single program for all dementia patients or whether different programs should be provided for persons with milder and more severe dementia. The answer to this question depends on the particular center and the individual participants. As dementia progresses, many patients become less able to participate in activity programs. Inability of the facility to adapt to this changing need is one reason leading to discharge from the day programs. We believe that programs which have the resources and an adequate number of participants function better with programs that vary activities based on the severity of the person's illness, but financial and size limitations often prevent the provision of more than one group at a time.

Group Homes and Assisted Living Facilities

In the past 10 years, there has been a rapid increase in the number of group home and assisted living facilities marketing themselves as appropriate for demented patients. These settings are often attractive because they look less institutional and almost always cost less than a traditional nursing home. As is the case with day centers, these environments are very diverse and are licensed differently in different states. Since licensure determines the amount of oversight that is provided by local health departments, this is an important issue. The frequent occurrence of dementia in these settings requires that group homes and assisted living facilities should have mechanisms in place to monitor mental health needs and to provide necessary care. Smaller group homes may lack structured activity programs and attendance at daycare should be considered if this is the case.

Nursing Homes

Sixty to 80% of individuals in nursing homes suffer from dementia. The principles and practices discussed in this book are universal and apply to the long-term-care setting as well as to dementia patients in the community. The residents of long-term-care facilities have a wide range of physical, social, behavioral, emotional, and cognitive impairments, and this presents a major challenge to the staff who provide care and design treatment programs. There is no convincing evidence that units labeled as *special care* for dementia patients are necessary to provide the appropriate level of stimulation and support for persons with dementia, but specific programs that address the activity, emotional, and physical needs of persons with dementia are needed. Special care units may be better able to care for the more seriously behaviorally impaired dementia patient but this has not been adequately demonstrated. Programs that address the need of the cognitively normal residents are also necessary. Staff training in caring for dementia patients and managing behavior is a critical aspect of care for any nursing home.

The Emergency Department

Acute changes in behavior or cognition are the most common reasons a patient with dementia is seen in an emergency department. Searching for an underlying physical cause of the behavior disturbance is crucial. History from knowledgeable informants can help the emergency team more quickly discover the cause or causes of the change in status. Atypical presentation of physical and psychiatric illness is common in the elderly, so lack of elevated temperatures and other signs of illness should not dissuade the team from a thorough evaluation. Treatment with sedatives or neuroleptics should be avoided if possible, until a cause has been identified or ruled out. Having someone who knows the patient stay with her at all times and repeating frequent explanations of what is happening can lessen the need for sedation.

The Acute Hospital

The majority of individuals in acute general hospitals are elderly. Individuals with dementia are prone to certain medical conditions which may lead to hospitalization. These conditions include delirium, hip fractures, arthritis, stroke, cancer, diabetes, hypertension, heart disease, and others. Therefore, it is no surprise that 6%–20% of persons over 65 in acute care hospitals suffer from dementia. Patients with dementia in the acute hospital should be monitored carefully for delirium due to medication intoxication, metabolic instability, or the complexities of their medical condition. Many will require constant reorientation and reminders about why they are in the hospital, what they should be doing, and what is planned for the future. If 24-hour support can be provided by family members or a nursing aide, it should be done before problems arise. If this is not possible, frequent brief interactions with staff should be used to remind and reorient patients. This will diminish patient distress and lessen problematic behaviors including wandering, climbing out of bed, and calling out. The prevalence of dementia is high enough that acute general hospitals should develop methods for identifying patients with dementia at the time of admission. This will improve the assessment and management of their special needs and improve the patients' and families' experiences in the hospital. It may also reduce the length of stay and the likelihood of restraint use. Since patients with dementia have average lengths of hospital stay 2–3 days longer than age-matched patients who are cognitively normal, this is an important issue.

Such a baseline assessment is especially important in same-day surgery centers.

Acute Psychiatric Units

The treatment of behavioral and mental disturbances in patients with dementia sometimes requires acute psychiatric hospitalization. Given the stigma associated with psychiatric treatment, it is best to mention the possibility of hospitalization to family members early in the treatment course if it is being considered. Because elderly patients with dementia have unique needs, they should be admitted to psychiatric units which have specifically trained, knowledgeable staff.

Hospice Care

Patients with late stage dementia who have been cared for at home are being referred for hospice care with increasing frequency (see Chapter 11). Hospice services are provided to persons having less than a 6-month life expectancy. This includes patients who are dependent, who are not eating and drinking, and whose families have agreed to forgo medical treatment of acute illnesses. Hospice care is sometimes provided at a designated hospice unit but sometimes the hospice team comes into the home and provides comfort measures for the patient and support for the family.

6

Supportive Care for
the Patient with Dementia

The goals of supportive care are to maintain quality of life and prevent morbidity. This chapter focuses on the general approach to the patient, issues in day-to-day living, safety and supervision, and health maintenance.

APPROACHING THE PATIENT

Establishing a Relationship

The first step in dementia care is forming a relationship with the patient. This begins with the initial contact, which should include time alone with the ill person to appreciate his experience of the illness. The situation of patients is best understood by taking into account their lives before the illness and the changes the illness has forced upon them.

One of the great challenges in caring for patients with dementia is maintaining their dignity as persons. This includes being sensitive to their feelings, adapting one's approach to their needs, and providing an environment as similar as possible to that previously experienced. Respecting the dignity of the individual involves not laughing at patients but laughing with them when the situation warrants. It involves understanding that privacy is desirable but recognizing that there are times when danger requires it be overridden. And it includes the responsibility to report to authorities any inappropriate conduct on the part of caregivers.

The time spent appreciating the life which has come before the illness helps the caregiver appreciate the patient's current emotional state and sets the stage for an empathic relationship throughout the course of the illness. In the early stages of dementia, many patients express fears about losing their abilities but most moderately to severely impaired patients have no appreciation of their impairment. This lack of insight is the result of the dementing illness and should not be viewed as psychological "denial." Therefore, we do not recommend arguing with individuals who have dementia when they make incorrect statements (for example, saying, "My mother is coming to pick me up" when she has been dead for years) or resist a medically necessary action such as taking medication or visiting the doctor. It is almost always better to empathize ("I'd be upset, too") or respond supportively ("While we're waiting could you help me"?) rather than confrontationally.

Communication

Impairments in communication are major impediments to establishing and maintaining a relationship. Patients with cortical dementias develop difficulties in making themselves understood (*expressive aphasia*) and in understanding others (*receptive aphasia*). They may substitute a word that sounds similar to the one they cannot remember. They may describe the function of an object they cannot name—for example, "I need the thing for drinking," instead of "I want my coffee cup." Many patients retain the rhythm, intonation, prosody, and gestures of speech long after they lose the ability to communicate with words. These aspects of speech are called the *pragmatics*.

Paying attention to the pragmatics of speech can enhance one's ability to understand what the patient is trying to say. Such was the case with a patient who only spoke in numbers. When greeted in the waiting room of the clinic with the words, "Good Morning, Mrs. Evans. How are you?" she would make eye contact, smile, reach out to shake hands, and respond, "Twenty-four, three seventy-one!" The pragmatics of her talk communicated that she was responding and telling the greeter she was fine. Prosody and pragmatics also help patients understand what is being said to them. Unfortunately, some caregivers use an approach which minimizes prosody. Raising one's voice and using a monotone to say, "How are you?" eliminates prosody and makes communication even more difficult.

Taking time to listen for key words can also help the clinician understand what patients are attempting to say. Some patients are embarrassed by difficulties in communication and become withdrawn from their families and from social groups. Careful listening and observation can re-moralize them and help them become more functional.

An issue over which there is disagreement among experts is whether patients should be addressed by first names or more formally ("Mr. X"). Some patients respond only to their first name. Many women with dementia forget their married name but respond to their maiden name. Therefore, the choice of using first or last names is a question that depends on the particular caregiver and patient. We suggest that clinicians introduce themselves as Mr., Ms., or Mrs._____ and address most patients by their last names. If the patient doesn't respond, the first name should be used. Some caregivers, particularly those who spend many hours with patients, are most comfortable and find patients most responsive when first names are used. This seems quite appropriate to us, particularly when the care providers use their own first names. For example, "Hi, Bill, it's Esther. Let's go down the hall and join the sing-along."

It is important to be cautious about the use of terms of endearment when speaking with patients. It is quite natural for husbands and wives to call each other 'honey' or 'sweetheart,' but it is rarely appropriate for a professional care provider (even an aide in a nursing home) to use that form of address with a patient. The use of such informal terms of endearment can be especially confusing to patients with dementia, who may respond "inkind" (inappropriately) or may feel frightened, overwhelmed, and unable to communicate their mistrust.

It is helpful to make eye contact before beginning to speak. Clinicians should ensure that patients can see and hear them by putting on the patients' eyeglasses and keeping hearing aids in working order. Dentures can help people speak more clearly. Bend down or kneel to speak to and maintain the attention of seated or lying patients. Gentle touch can gain and maintain the attention of a patient who is easily distracted. Other noise and distraction should be kept to a minimum, and radios and televisions should be turned off.

Clinicians should ask only one question at a time and give the patient time to respond. Patients with Parkinson disease, Huntington disease, and other subcortical dementias often need more time. If English is a second language, patients often revert to their first language as they become more impaired. Clinicians should speak slowly and use short, uncomplicated sentences. If patients are struggling to find a word, the clinician should offer a guess.

Directions that are given one step at a time will improve the ability of the patient to understand and cooperate. If the person doesn't seem to understand directions, a gesture may be given. Clinicians should use nouns and names frequently. When speaking about a third person, use the name rather than "he" or "she". Similarly, use nouns when possible. For example, ask, "Do you want cake?" rather than, "Do you want it?" A positive approach to communication is usually more helpful than a negative one. For example, when patients attempt to leave a safe area, they will respond more readily to an invitation to engage in a pleasant activity than to being told, "You can't go out there."

Nonverbal communication becomes increasingly important as the dementia progresses. Caregivers pay even more attention to facial expressions and gestures, and patients will respond to a smile and a gentle touch even if they cannot understand any words. When patients do not seem to understand something, the care-provider should try to regain their attention and speak slowly and quietly rather than more loudly. These general steps in successful communication are summarized in Table 6.1.

SUPPORT IN DAY-TO-DAY LIVING

Maximizing Function and Identifying Abilities

The day-to-day living of patients should be structured to maximize their remaining abilities and function. This preserves their dignity, makes life easier for caregivers, and possibly encourages abilities to persist for longer periods of time. Clinicians should work with caregivers to find settings and environments in which limitations are minimized and remaining abilities are maximized.

When structuring the day-to-day living of patients, the clinician should consider their prior interests, wishes, and usual activity level. Among the questions to be asked are: Were they someone who was al-

Table 6.1. Tips for Communicating with Language-Impaired Patients

Addressing the Patient	Responding to the Patient
1. Address the patient by name and identify yourself	1. Listen for key words
2. Make eye contact; sit or kneel for seated patients	2. Observe and respond to the emotional tone of the communication
3. Reduce distractions: turn off the radio and television	3. Observe and interpret body language, rhythm, and rate of speech
4. Make sure the patient is using eyeglasses and functioning hearing aids	4. Offer a guess
5. Speak slowly in a low tone of voice. Give commands one step at a time. Use visual cues and gentle physical guidance when needed	

ways active with other people or did they typically do things in small groups or alone? What sorts of specific things did they like to do? How did they pace and structure their life? In what ways did they derive pleasure and enjoyment? How important were routines and predictability?

One difficult aspect of maximizing function is the fluctuating nature of some patients' abilities. They may be able to do some of their activities one day but may resist and be overwhelmed by it on another. Sometimes, these fluctuations can be explained by environmental, medical, or psychological events, but usually a specific cause is not identified. Thus, the maximization of function is an important goal, but is not always possible to accomplish.

Periodic reassessment is important. As impairments accumulate, it can be helpful to focus on activities and functions that remain of interest to the patient. For example, patients who are able to perform basic activities of daily living (ADLs) but show limited interests in participating in other activities would be more active if their day were structured around ADLs.

A Place to Live

A variety of living arrangements and environments is available for patients with dementia. Early in the disease, most continue to live in their homes. Others move into the homes of their children, either fully integrated, or in special living spaces which the children develop for them, such as additions or renovated basements or attics. Some patients may live in assisted living environments. Assisted living is becoming increasingly available in the United States. It provides meals and some direction but requires that the person be able to take medication on their own. Facilities range from small "Mom and Pop" operations, usually housing a small number (fewer than 5–10) of individuals who may have dementia, to larger, more institutional operations. Finally, there are nursing homes and skilled nursing facilities where dementia patients may reside, either integrated with residents who require general nursing care or in special areas designed for the care of dementia (special care units). The best place for individuals is determined by their level of functioning and their available resources.

A common question that usually arises early in the course of dementia is whether the patient is able to live alone. This is possible for individuals who can perform their daily living activities well, can safely provide their own nutrition, hydration, and basic activities, and know what to do if an emergency arises. If there is any doubt about a patient's ability to live independently, an assessment by an occupational therapist can provide useful information. Some patients are able to live alone safely for a period of time if they are provided help with meal preparation and medication supervision and are checked regularly by telephone or in person. Participation in an activity program out of the home, such as a senior citizen center or adult day program, can prolong their ability to live independently. Patients who are not able to live alone might do well if they have a companion living with them. This could be a family member or a hired aide. Many individuals move in with children or other family members.

Patients with dementia require environments that are safe, stable, and able to accommodate to their cognitive, functional, behavioral, and medical impairments. The environment should be neat and clutter free, because this enhances the ability of the patient to focus on the task at hand. For example, a dining room table that has only a place setting on a contrasting table mat is preferable to a table that has newspapers, daily mail, and toys. Likewise, a bathroom sink that only has a toothbrush and toothpaste visible enables the ill person to pay attention to these specific cues rather than to bottles, lotions, laundry, and other objects. Photographs and familiar objects throughout the house or in a room provide many cues and orient the patient to his/her past life.

Nutrition and Hydration

Maintenance of adequate nutrition and hydration can be a challenge for several reasons. Dementia impairs the ability to plan and prepare meals, to differentiate fresh from spoiled foods, to eat a balanced diet, or to remember to eat at all. Because these impairments are common, meals often must be organized and monitored by the caregiver. Inedible garnishes should not be used and decorative wax or plastic fruits should be eliminated from the home. It is better for the caregiver to offer condiments to the patient rather than leave them on the table.

The dignity of the patient can be preserved by preparing plates of food in the kitchen and cutting that food away from the view of others. Many foods can be prepared to be eaten as finger food for patients who can no longer use utensils. Tough meat should be avoided. Since some patients eat rapidly and choke, the caregiver should learn how to perform the Heimlich maneuver. Small amounts of food can be offered gradually to avoid gorging. Weekly or monthly weigh-ins can be used to monitor intake and identify weight problems earlier.

Fluid intake should be monitored carefully. Patients may misidentify a dangerous liquid, such as a cleaner or paint, and drink it when thirsty. In order to ensure adequate intake, fluids should be offered every 2 hours. Caffeinated beverages should be avoided and fluid limited in the evening to minimize nighttime awakenings caused by the need to void.

Sleep Hygiene

Adequate rest is an important factor in assuring optimal functioning. Day–night sleep cycles can be easily disturbed and even reversed in dementia. Establishing a routine of activities leading up to bedtime will facilitate adequate rest. Daily exercise and exposure to bright light (at times through bright light devices) can assist in maintaining normal sleep cycles. Keeping the patient awake in the evening is a challenge for many families. Scheduling evening activities that patients enjoy can prevent them from wanting to go to bed too early. When complaints about sleep are raised, caregivers should be asked to monitor total sleep in a 24 hour diary. The patient who naps on and off during the day often needs less sleep at night and resists going to bed at night. Keeping patients dressed during the day and in bedclothes at the same time each night can further cue the patient that he should be preparing for sleep.

The temperature of the bedroom should be comfortable and night clothing should be loose fitting. Night-lights are helpful to some patients, but the shadows that result can be frightening. Some medications, including beta-blockers and antidepressants, can cause frightening dreams that disturb sleep. Sleep medications should be avoided, if possible, as they can impair the sleep–wake cycle and cause increased confusion. Further discussion of management of sleep disturbance is in Chapter 9.

Establishing a Daily Routine

Because the dementias rob people of flexibility and adaptability, the vast majority of patients do better in a stable, predictable environment, even very early in the illness. Ideally, these routines should be patterned after those that the patient and family followed for years. There are plausible reasons why a stable, unchanging routine is helpful and supportive to many people with dementia. First, a predictable pattern of activity is likely to maximize the ability to learn. The more routines are repeated and the more they are reinforced by the environment, the greater the likelihood that the patient will learn. For example, many patients learn where the bathroom is several weeks or months after moving into a nursing home, presumably because of repetition. A second reason that daily routines help patients is that they provide predictability. If patients associate taking medication with mealtime, for example, they are more likely to learn that they will eat right after they take their medicine and to be more cooperative with both.

Establishing a predictable and repetitive routine is not always easy. Activities and situations can change and necessitate an alteration in schedules. Conversely, the goal of establishing regularity should not prevent the development of new activities or routines. This is important since the maintenance of an interesting and stimulating life sometimes requires the introduction of new activities. Ideally, new activities will draw upon previously learned and enjoyed activities. For example, holiday parties in nursing homes generate the same kind of excitement that they do at home or among schoolchildren in the classroom. Some of this excitement comes from staff and families, but patients also get caught up in the fun because holidays involve rituals and behaviors that have been lifelong. Even very impaired individuals can participate and actively enjoy the excitement and pleasures of celebrations.

Successful Activities

Activities should stimulate as many of the patient's remaining capacities as possible. They provide pleasure, keep people occupied, strengthen muscles, and help people feel useful. Getting dressed and making the bed are activities and opportunities for success as much as a ball toss or arm stretching. With activities viewed in this way, time can be organized to make life pleasurable and meaningful for both the patient and caregiver.

Family members often ask how to determine if an activity is a "success" or not. The outcome to look for is interest and involvement on the part of the patient. For patients who are very impaired and who have limited attention spans, simply being in a room with others and observing an activity such as dinner preparation may be enjoyable and convey that they are still part of the family. Even though patients may not recall an activity or event later, they can enjoy it while it is occurring.

Providing activities for a person with dementia can be very time consuming. We suggest that a schedule of activities be written down on a calendar and put in a prominent place such as on the refrigerator. A written plan will also assist in continuity when more than one caregiver is involved. Having a scheduled routine can also help caregivers by allowing them to set aside times to attend their own needs.

Emotional Support

Patients with dementia have the same need for emotional support as any other person. This need increases when difficulties with day-to-day living are encountered or when bad news such as the illness or death of a friend or spouse is learned. Emotional support may take the form of spending more time with the ill person, encouraging them and listening to their distress. Occasionally, professional support in the form of individual counseling or group psychotherapy is necessary. Patients with milder dementia are better able to benefit from these sorts of professional interventions. In institutional settings such as assisted living and nursing homes, the need for emotional support can get lost in the rigid structure of the institutional routine because the caregivers and professionals do not have much time to sit and listen.

However, many patients with dementia are aware that they are losing their memory and ability to think and become distressed. These feelings should be directly addressed by acknowledging their upset, validating the source of the distress, and encouraging them to refocus their thinking on things that they can accomplish. Establishing tasks and goals that can be accomplished, implementing them, and having successes over a period of time are important steps in re-moralizing patients with dementia who feel that they are losing the ability to control themselves and their environment.

Some patients with dementia will be upset by anticipating the future. Again, support can be provided by allowing them to express their thoughts and feelings, providing emotional support, helping them identify and maintain positive aspects of their lives, and providing information about the ability to preserve and maintain dignity even with advanced dementia. Clinicians in any environment and of any professional background can provide this support to dementia patients.

Travel

Travel may be desired or necessary for many reasons: visiting family, moving closer to family, or continuing regular travel that has been part of the couple's retirement plans. Significant events that occur in the patient's life such as weddings, graduations, and funerals may require traveling long distances.

Unfortunately, travel with a person who has dementia can be quite difficult. Nevertheless, it is possible, even in advanced stages, if the appropriate steps are taken. First, start by deciding if the travel is necessary or beneficial for the patient. For example, a visit to a recently born grandchild can directly benefit patients who have the capacity to appreciate the event. However, a spouse may wish to take a patient on a cruise but not realize that the patient has lost the ability to enjoy the cruise.

Once it is clear that travel can be beneficial to the patient and that the patient wants to go, consider the means of travel. It is best to travel the fastest way (usually by airplane), to travel to as familiar an environment as possible, and to provide distraction and personal time for the patient during the trip. If a patient is to travel by air, inform the airline that a dementia patient will be traveling. Most airlines will provide preferential seating to dementia patients; for example, close to the bathroom or on the aisle with more leg room. They can be escorted onto the airplane earlier than other passengers and be given wheelchair assistance if needed.

During travel, minimize what is expected of the patient. Luggage should be taken care of by the person accompanying the patient. Driving to and from airports and train stations should be limited as much as possible by using the closest and quickest destination. Scheduling travel for times that are least busy such as late in the day or on Saturdays can lessen overstimulation.

During the trip, make sure that the patient remains adequately hydrated and fed. Planned activities—for example, being read to, listening to a portable tape player, or playing a card game—can distract and engage the ill person. After arrival it is better to rest and relax rather than immediately become involved in another exciting or stressful activity. One-on-one attention from a familiar person is ideal. If travel across time zones is involved, the family should talk to their physician about use of a sedative-hypnotic pill that will help the patient sleep upon arrival.

Out of Home Placement

Patients who are unable to live alone or whose spouse or children cannot provide care are candidates for moving into an organized, supported living situation. This is referred to as *placement* and can be particularly difficult for family caregivers, since placement is often lifelong. Some caregivers see placement as a failure on their part but we see it as a necessary step for many individuals because of the impairments caused by the disease.

The need for placement usually results from one of four reasons. First, patients' cognitive impairment may be such that they are no longer able to recognize or interact with their environment. Second, functional decline may cause them to be dependent on others. Impairments in dressing, bathing, feeding, toileting, and ambulating are major reasons for placement. The development of chronic behavioral disturbances that are hard to treat or manage and that require constant supervision is a third common reason for placement. Finally, there are comorbid medical disorders which require specialized nursing care. Table 6.2 lists some of the factors that necessitate long term care placement.

The transition between living situations is an important aspect of supportive care. If patients need to move out of their house, no longer live alone, or are about to be placed in assisted living or a nursing home, they will face a period of adjustment. They usually have little say in such transitions, although most will go along with them because others tell them that it is appropriate. When possible, transitions should be

Table 6.2. Common Reasons for Out of Home Placement in Dementia

Patient Factors	Family and Resource Factors
Need for 24 hour supervision, e.g., due to wandering	Lack of available caregiver
Aggression during care on a regular basis	Caregiver is impaired: frail, depressed,
Dependence on others for basic, living activities such as eating	Death of primary caregiver
Complex comorbid medical illnesses	Respite unavailable for caregiver: cannot afford daycare or assistance, other family member not available
Unpredictable behavior	Unsuitable home or caregiving location
Constant pacing	
Confinement to bed	

planned well ahead of time so that they can take place in an organized fashion. If the patient's level of insight and ability to appreciate the need for the transition is impaired, it is usually necessary to limit their involvement in planning and executing the transition. (See discussion in Chapter 12 regarding the ethical issues that this raises.)

Unanimity among family members and clinicians can make a move smoother. Patients who cannot appreciate the need to move may do better if the time period that they have to brood or worry over the move is limited. On occasion, it is best if the patient is not told about the move until the last minute.

Preparation of the new environment is important. Whether moving into the home of a relative or an institution, having familiar objects in sight and regular routines established can smooth the transition. Many individuals benefit from a tour of the facility before the move, but in some instances this is more upsetting.

For some patients, having frequent visitors is calming and positive. For others, however, it is better to limit visits until the patient becomes adjusted to the new environment and new staff. Some patients who move into new settings have difficulty sleeping at night and benefit from a sedative hypnotic medicine for a short period of time (typically less than a week). This can prevent disruption of the sleep–wake cycle during the transition. Most patients who move are able to adjust within a month. If adjustments problems last longer, an alternative explanation should be sought since new behavioral disturbances or medical disorders can cause similar problems.

SAFETY AND SUPERVISION

Several safety issues must be addressed in caring for a dementia patient. Driving and falls are discussed in Chapter 9 and will not be considered here.

Household accidents are common. Some are minor and unrelated to having dementia, but most are caused by the dementia. Some result from loss of memory—for example, leaving the stove on, allowing food to spoil out of the refrigerator and eating it anyway, or forgetting to lock doors.

Wandering and getting lost are serious problems which need to be considered in every patient at every point in the illness. At the very least, all patients should wear an identification bracelet which provides name, address, and emergency phone number.

Smoking is less prevalent than in the past but is still an issue. Whenever possible, efforts should be made to help the patient quit. If total abstinence from smoking is not possible, then observation during smoking is necessary. Hunting and access to weapons is problematic in some areas. Like driving, hunting is an activity that has often been lifelong and symbolic of achieving independence. Finally, financial and personal victimization, particularly in patients who maintain their finances or who are left at home unsupervised, can also be problematic. Limiting the control that patients have over their assets is often the best protection.

Prevention and Safety-Proofing

In the home. One of the challenges in caring for patients with dementia is making the environment safe *before* an accident happens. Families should be told that patients can be unpredictable and do things they would not have done before becoming ill. Even though they can still read labels on containers, patients lose the ability to sense what is appropriate to eat or drink and what is unsafe. Because of visual agnosia, patients lose the ability to see hazards around them. They are at risk of climbing out of an upper story window or over the safety rails on a bed or of wandering out into traffic. Many patients will not recognize the significance of a car horn, smoke detector alarm, or the smell of smoke. They are at risk of scalding themselves if they lose the ability to regulate water temperature appropriately prior to taking a bath. Adequate lighting can increase the ability of patients to perceive what is around them. Stairwells should be brightly lit, day and night, as should doorways to the bathroom. Handrails on stairs must be secured into the studs to prevent a patient from pulling them out, thus possibly falling and becoming injured. Exposed radiators and hot water pipes should be insulated to prevent their burning the patient who touches them or sits on them.

Baby gates across stairwells and doorways are only useful if they prevent the patient from crawling under or climbing over them. Many families use two baby gates to prevent a patient from entering an area which would be unsafe. Inexpensive motion sensors can be placed to alert a caregiver to when patients attempt to enter a room where they should not be or to when they get up at night and need to be escorted to the bathroom and back to bed.

Clinicians must assume that a dementia patient may eat or fiddle with anything. Potentially toxic plants should be removed from the environment, cleaning solutions should be kept under lock and key, and power tools should be locked up and kept inaccessible to the patient. Even salt and pepper shakers may need to be removed and put out of sight. We have known patients to eat their hearing aids, flowers, and a bowl of shells (perhaps perceiving it as a bowl of snack food) and to drink a bottle of paint (perhaps thinking it was fruit punch).

It is essential that patients wear identification such as a bracelet or pendant on a necklace. These are available through Medic Alert and the Alzheimer's Association. They can be made attractive for persons who are bothered by the appearance of such items. Keeping a recent photograph readily available at all times will aid in finding an individual who gets lost. People who are agnosic and anxious may need only a moment of turning away from their care provider to become frightened and rapidly walk away. Putting labels in clothing can help identify a person who does not have a wallet or purse. One creative family whose grandfather wore a baseball cap put his last name in bold letters on his baseball cap so he could be easily identified if he wandered away at a county fair.

Patients may not perceive hazards in front of them and trip on them. In the home, clutter should be eliminated, rugs should be tacked down securely, and low pieces of furniture that the patient may not notice should be removed. For patients who have a diminished perception of depth, a contrasting strip of tape on the edge of steps may increase contrast or depth perception and help the patient see the edge. Obviously, swimming pools should be securely fenced and the patient should not be able to get to ponds or streams.

Cigarettes, cigars, pipes, and matches must be secured in a locked cabinet away from patients and their use should be supervised at all times. Gas or electric stoves should be turned off to prevent a patient from attempting to light a cigarette on the burner.

A NO SOLICITATIONS sign on the door may be helpful in keeping salesmen away from the home. However, the best protection from financial victimization is to limit the patient's access to money, bank accounts, and other resources.

Bathrooms can be hazardous in many ways. Medications, razors, bars of soap, and scissors should be secured away from the patient's view and access. A bath mat is essential to prevent falling on a slippery wet floor. Urine and water must be wiped up immediately to prevent falls. It is important to turn the thermostat down on the hot water heater so that patients cannot scald themselves. Caregivers should either reverse or remove bathroom locks or tape open the bathroom door so that the patients don't lock themselves in. Windows should be securely locked or only be able to be opened 6 inches to prevent patients from crawling out. Pullcords on shades, blinds, and draperies should be pulled up and secured out of the view of the patient, and electric cords must be securely tacked down.

In the kitchen, families can have a master switch installed on the stove so they can turn it off when unsupervised. Similarly, coffee pots and irons that have an automatic shutoff can be invaluable. Sharp instruments such as carving knives should be stored out of sight or locked away. Families must be vigilant in observing what is in the refrigerator of patients who live on their own since they may lose the ability to determine which food is fresh and which food is spoiled.

In the nursing home and other institutional settings. The same cautions apply in long term care settings. The potential to ingest harmful substances is a particular hazard. All staff, including housekeeping, must be educated to assure that hazardous substances, whether cleaning supplies or condiments, are not available to patients. Thus, items such as bottles of Betadine and craft paint must be kept away from the patients. Supplies in arts and crafts classes, including magic markers, must be nontoxic. Electric socket covers, such as those used in childproofing, are useful in preventing electric shock; those that are clear plastic will be much more difficult for patients to remove.

Items such as shaving cream and razors (whether blade or electric) should not be left in patients' rooms. Additionally, rooms in a nursing home should be routinely examined to see if the residents are hoarding food that can become spoiled. Windows should be stopped at 6 inches to avoid a patient going out through them. In outdoor areas, protective fences should be high enough to prevent patients from climbing over or being boosted over by other patients. Garden furniture should be heavy so that it cannot be moved to a wall to be used as a climbing aid.

Motion sensors and key padlocked doors are very useful in nursing homes, as are wander guards (a bracelet that triggers an alarm when the patient leaves the area). Low flat-heel shoes that are the right size will aid greatly in gait stability. Conversely, sashes that hang down or pants that are too long will place a patient at increased risk for falls. Remove items from pockets of patients' clothing before laundering since patients have been known to eat shredded paper and other substances after they have gone through the washing machine.

Patients who have full or partial dentures are particularly at risk for choking because bread or other soft foods can become entangled in the denture, leading patients to attempt to swallow them. Patients who eat very rapidly should have their food cut into small pieces before serving and be kept away from other persons' dinner plates. Pacing the rate at which food is presented can avoid choking. Staff should be trained in the Heimlich maneuver in the event that a patient chokes. Ornaments placed on holiday decorations such as a Christmas tree should be made of edible substances such as cookie dough or a string of licorice with Fruit Loops on it. Christmas lights should be eliminated. At other holidays, such as Easter, decorations that might be perceived as edible should be edible. Real or candy eggs are safer than plastic or paper mache decorations, for example.

If patients persistently try to leave a facility, it is preferable to place them in a secure setting such as a locked area/unit rather than to sedate or restrain them. Patients need sufficient space to wander about safely and restraints are not an acceptable alternative to a safe environment. Bed rails are generally hazardous to patients with dementia since they often try to climb over them.

Leaving Patients Alone

Given the wide-ranging safety concerns discussed above and the fact that safety-proofing does not always prevent problems, it is reasonable to ask whether any individual with dementia can be left alone. Clearly, in more advanced dementia, patients cannot be left alone because they are at high risk of harm. However, for many patients, some degree of independence is desirable as this maintains dignity, privacy, and quality of life. These benefits must be balanced against the risks of being left alone. Rather than all or nothing, this is often best viewed as a graded issue: Some patients can be left alone for part of the time or with limited supervision. Table 6.3 provides a list of questions to ask when determining whether an individual should be left alone.

MAINTAINING HEALTH

Purpose and Coordination

Patients with dementia are susceptible to developing delirium in response to minor changes in their physical homeostasis and are vulnerable to becoming upset, distressed, or explosive in reaction to what appears to be a small or minor discomfort.

Table 6.3. Should Patients Be Left Alone?

If You Answer NO to Any of the Following Questions, the Person Should Not Be Left Alone
1. Can they make phone calls?
2. Can they tell you their full name, address, directions to their house, telephone number?
3. Can they tell you what they would do if a fire started?
4. Can they tell you what they would do if they fell down or became suddenly ill?
5. Can they identify persons who should be allowed to enter the house and those who should not?

If You Answer YES to Any of the Following, the Person Should Not Be Left Alone
1. Does the patient say they "want to go home" when they are home?
2. Have they wandered out of the house?
3. Have they been lost in the neighborhood?
4. Do they ever misidentify you or members of the family?
5. Do they smoke cigarettes, pipes, or cigars?

Unfortunately, most patients with dementia are not able to coordinate their own health care and must rely on a caregiver for help. It is important that each patient have a primary care physician who has an understanding of dementia and can respond to acute changes in the patient's physical and behavioral status. The caregiver should know the medical diagnosis of the patient and a knowledge of the medicines that they take, including dose frequency, administration route, purpose, and potential side effects.

Basic Hygiene and Preventive Care

The maintenance of good dental health presents a major challenge. Early in the course of dementia, many patients lose the ability to perform adequate oral hygiene and need help brushing and flossing daily. Patients should have their teeth cleaned every 3 to 6 months at the dental office. These cleanings offer the opportunity for close inspection of teeth and gum conditions. As the dementia progresses, the need for vigilant inspection increases since resistance to routine care often results in broken teeth, abscesses, and dental caries.

Denture care is also important. Patients with dentures may forget to insert them properly or to clean them. Having a routine place to soak them at night and supervision for insertion in the morning will minimize the chance for loss of dentures. Proper insertion with appropriate adhesives will also ensure that eating is comfortable and lessen the likelihood that they will be thrown away. Proper-fitting dentures also allow appropriate appearance and speech.

Preventive care also includes attention to the skin and feet, most easily done during bathing. Caregivers should inspect patients' skin for any erosions, rashes, or bruises. These may indicate malfitting clothing or previous falls. Any redness in a skin fold can cause discomfort and can be treated with cornstarch. During winter, lotions should be applied to the skin to prevent dryness and itching. Periodic podiatric care can assure that feet are free from infection and that nails are appropriately cut. The gentle application of lotions to the skin and feet also provide a source of pleasure and relaxation for patients.

Attention to hearing and vision will assure that patients can function maximally. Glasses should be kept clean and worn with a cord to secure them. Hearing aids should be kept in working order and put away at night.

Careful attention to elimination patterns is also important. Patients may not complain of trouble passing their water or moving their bowels due to forgetfulness or poor judgment. The caregiver should monitor bowel movements and ensure their occurrence at least two or three times per week. Stool softeners or other medications may be necessary if dietary regulation does not assure regular bowel movements. Caregivers should also monitor for bladder infections whose only sign may be increased confusion, unexpected incontinence, or frequent bathroom use.

Other aspects of preventive care include the monitoring of comorbid chronic illnesses and annual visits to the primary physician for flu shots, mammograms, Pap tests, and prostate exams. Caregivers should be encouraged to participate in the visits to provide information and to record any instructions.

Medication Administration

The primary caregiver should take responsibility for medication administration since the risk of patients' forgetting to take prescribed medications and the risk of taking too much because they have forgotten are high. As is the case for any older person, the medication regime should be organized so that only essential medicines are given and on a schedule which is acceptable to the patient. A dosing schedule which minimizes the number of times the medication needs to be given is ideal. Given the many demands of caregiving, many family members use a calendar to check off when medications are given. Because of the potential for accidental misuse, medications, including over-the-counter drugs, should be kept safely out of the reach of patients. Child-guard caps may not be sufficient to ensure that patients do not open the bottles.

Some patients may resist taking medications or have difficulty swallowing pills. Caregivers may need to be taught how to crush medications and disguise them in pudding, applesauce, ice cream, or other sweet foods the patient will accept, but they should check with the physician to make sure that this is appropriate. Medications that are available in a liquid form are often easier to administer. Optimally, such medications should be given with food as part of a meal, thus minimizing the need to convince patients to take them. This is especially helpful with patients who are suspicious that their medications have been tampered with.

Procedures/Surgery

In general, dementia is not a contraindication for any operation. However, it is important for any dementia patient and/or caregiver to consider the risk–benefit equation prior to agreeing to an operation. It is important to determine the purpose for which any procedure is being done, as well as its potential risks and benefits. The impact the dementia may have on choosing to have the procedure or on managing the patient after the procedure should be explicitly discussed. For example, patients with very advanced dementia who are preterminal and have symptoms of cancer might not be a candidate for a CT scan of their chest if nothing would be done to treat their cancer. The potential benefit to patients needs to be weighed carefully. We have had one patient with very advanced dementia who had prolapse of the uterus into the vagina and developed the belief that she was pregnant, which was very distressing to her. The problem was resolved after a successful vaginal hysterectomy.

Once the decision has been made to proceed with a procedure or operation, it is important to focus on reducing the adverse effects of the procedure by using anesthetic agents with as short a half life as possible and by minimizing medication and restraint during recovery.

If major surgery is being contemplated, it may be wise to ask the dementia care specialist to discuss the matter with the surgeon and anesthesiologist. Additionally, it is important to appreciate that postoperatively, after even minor procedures, many dementia patients develop a delirium that can last several days. The best way to address this is to provide one-on-one supervision by a familiar person throughout the hospital stay. It is important to attempt to avoid restraints, to be reassuring, and to use medications judiciously, as these may prolong delirium. The section on delirium in Chapter 8 provides information about the management of a delirium.

7

Supporting the Family and the Care-Provider

*T*he day-to-day caregiver of the person with dementia, whether a family member, friend, or professional, is her lifeline to the world around. No treatment plan is complete without a good understanding of who caregivers are and what they are facing, and without intervention to help the caregiver. This chapter discusses these matters in detail.

THE FAMILY CAREGIVER

More than two-thirds of people with dementia live at home and the majority are cared for by family members. Compared to people who live at home, individuals living in long-term-care facilities are more physically ill, more frail, older, less likely to have the ability to feed and dress themselves, and less likely to have living relatives. These differences demonstrate that many individuals are admitted to nursing homes because their family can no longer provide the level of care they need or because there is no one else available to provide care. The average age of caregivers is 57 years. This highlights the fact that the spouse caregivers are also elderly and that daughters and daughters-in-law may also be employed and have responsibilities for their own nuclear families.

Who are the care-providers for the elderly still living at home? In the United States most are women. About half are wives and another third are daughters or daughters-in-law. Husbands provide 10% of the care;

the remainder is provided by other relatives such as sons, nieces, and nephews, or by hired aides.

Much of what we know about family care-providers comes from people who have taken a relative to a dementia evaluation clinic or who have joined a family support group. Many individuals who care for someone with dementia at home have not sought help from a medical or social service professional or from informal support groups. Since caregivers who have been studied are probably quite different from those who have not sought professional attention for their relative or themselves, we know little about the concerns and needs of many caregivers.

Providing care for a person with dementia is both rewarding and stressful. We tend to hear little about the rewards and a great deal about the stresses. In this chapter we will emphasize the problems that caregivers have, because this is a book about helping distressed or ill individuals. It is important to remember, though, that many (probably the majority) care-providers are doing well emotionally. In one study done by our group, more than 60% of families did not report significant emotional distress. Therefore, a majority of caregivers may not require any type of assistance beyond that which they have been able to obtain themselves through family, friends, social service agencies, hired individuals, community resources (such as day care centers), or a health professional.

HOW COMMON IS DISTRESS IN CAREGIVERS?

More than one-third of families who join a family support group or have their relatives cared for in a dementia center are experiencing significant levels of emotional distress. This has been demonstrated in many studies using many different methods. Studies that measure depression or distress in caregivers report that rates of these symptoms are two to three times higher in dementia caregivers than in the general population. Other studies have shown that tranquilizer and sedative use is higher among caregivers than in the general population. Still others reveal that social isolation and family disagreements are more prevalent than in similar families who are not caring for someone with dementia.

What kinds of emotional problems do caregivers have? The majority of those who are distressed experience a mixture of feelings: Frustration, anger, sadness, and irritability are all common. Often these feelings fluctuate and depend on how well things are going that day or week. Twenty percent of caregivers in some studies report that distress is present much of every day. Many caregivers also report feeling physically exhausted, having difficulty sleeping, or lacking their normal level of energy. It is not easy to decide whether these feelings result from overwork or demoralization, but it is likely that both contribute. Research has not demonstrated that care providers have poorer physical health than the population at large though many believe that this is the case. Clearly, ill health is a common reason for caregivers to stop providing direct care for an ill person.

Surprisingly, the few studies which have followed caregivers over time have found that they tend to do *better* emotionally over time even though the dementia becomes more severe. This finding suggests that many people can utilize their innate psychological strengths and external social and financial supports in times of difficulty to adapt to and overcome many problems. Caregivers likely have more needs than others, but most do not need constant emotional, physical, and social assistance. The following paragraphs discuss, in more detail, some of the negative feelings that caregiving engenders. As already stated, these feelings frequently coexist and often fluctuate, depending upon the circumstances of the moment.

Grief

Many professionals who help caregivers have talked about grief as a way of understanding the emotional experiences of family carers. The word *grief* refers to the universal human emotional state that accompanies the loss of a person or object that is important to the individual. Grief is characterized by a variety of feelings that come and go. Sadness is the emotion that most people associate with grieving and it usually comes on suddenly ("a welling up of grief") when the person is reminded of the person or thing which has been lost. In the grief associated with the death of a loved one, physical symptoms such as difficulty falling asleep, low energy, and diminished appetite are common.

Studies show that the majority of grieving individuals report significant diminution in these symptoms by 3 months after the death of a loved one. However, even after a year, intermittent sadness is common, usually brought on by reminders of the deceased person. It is common for a photograph, special object, or anniversary to trigger a memory of the deceased and rekindle the feeling of loss.

Another aspect of grief that is well known through the writings of Elizabeth Kubler-Ross, Murray Parkes, and others is that grief follows a typical course. Numbness and anger are common in the early phases of grief; acceptance usually emerges later, often after several months. It is important to note, however, that these feeling states intermingle and do not occur in specific, time-limited, sequential steps.

Emotional experiences similar to those seen in grief are reported by *some* caregivers. This has led some to speculate that caregivers experience *chronic grief*. Research to date has shown that caregivers, as a group, remain distressed over many years, but no study has found that there is a consistent pattern to this emotional distress. Anger and guilt appear to diminish over time in many caregivers but some individuals report that they adapt emotionally to one set of symptoms only to again become demoralized when a new set of disabilities or symptoms develops in their loved ones. This fluctuating roller-coaster of feelings is similar to the emotional state of acute grief. Thus, some caregivers do experience a state similar to chronic grief even though the ill person is not deceased. Supportive counseling is likely to benefit individuals who experience this chronic form of grief.

Anger

Anger is a common experience of caregivers. Many report that they have been frustrated, angry, and irritated with the ill person, the disease, friends, and family members. Anger can also be directed at professionals, institutions, or society. Some caregivers are embarrassed or distressed by this anger. Knowing that it is not only common but almost universal emphasizes that it is an understandable response to a sad, frustrating, uncomfortable, and unfair situation. Anger commonly arises around loyalty conflicts. This is the case when there have been several marriages. For example, if the caregiver has been married to the ill person only a short time, commitment to provide care may be uncertain. In addition, children from separate unions may not feel it is their compelling responsibility to step in and help.

Anger can have an undesirable or dangerous side. If expressed physically, it can lead to physical, psychological, or financial abuse of the ill person. Anger can also be expressed by neglect, thus placing the ill person at risk of harm. If unexpressed, it may increase the emotional turmoil experienced by the caregiver. Therefore, it is important to help caregivers appreciate that *frequent frustration and anger are warning signs of being overwhelmed*. Caregivers who are experiencing more than occasional anger outbursts should seek help. Acceptable settings in which these feelings can be expressed include discussions with friends or families, support groups, and counseling sessions with clergy or health professionals. Relief from some direct caregiving responsibilities (sometimes called *respite*) by paid professionals, family members, or friends is also helpful in reducing anger. A combination of these may be most beneficial.

Demoralization

The words *sadness, depression, discouragement, and demoralization* are often used interchangeably to describe an unhappy mood state. Unfortunately, the word *depression* has several meanings that are sometimes confused. *Depression* as in *clinical depression* is used by professionals to refer to a condition such as major depression or manic depressive illness in which the mood takes on a life of its own. In this type of depression individuals are sad almost every minute of the day for weeks or months. This low mood is often accompanied by feelings of low energy, decreased appetite, poor sleep, and self-deprecatory beliefs. This type of depression is uncommon in dementia caregivers. It will be referred to here as *clinical* depression to distinguish it from other depressed states.

Demoralization, in contrast, is a feeling of sinking low mood, upset, and distress that occurs when facing a problem without an easy solution. Almost all individuals have been demoralized at some point in their lives. Demoralization can be brief or long lasting and is often accompanied by a feeling of loss of control over circumstances. Many caregivers report feeling demoralized by the caregiving situation. A common comment is, "The future only holds more decline. There is nothing to look forward to."

Demoralized feelings usually fluctuate and are worse when caregiving becomes more frustrating. These feelings of discouragement often intermingle with the belief that things are going well or as well as they could be. Indeed, we suspect that caregivers who claim that they have never been discouraged by caregiving are either unaware of these feelings or fooling themselves. Research suggests that being able to talk about frustration and distress with a close friend or relative (sometimes called a *confidante*) is one important way in which many people get through periods of demoralization. It is probably for this reason that many caregivers do not require any specific professional, ministerial, or outside help even though demoralization and discouragement are universal feelings and are probably unavoidable when providing care for a person with dementia. Individuals who experience persistent demoralization should seek help. Support groups, pastoral counseling, professional counseling, respite, vacations, and hobbies are resources that can relieve or diminish the hopelessness that accompanies demoralization.

Some individuals realize on their own that they are becoming discouraged, demoralized, and frustrated and that they likely need to use available resources better or find additional ones. However, others do not see that their current emotional state is a problem. When this is the case, a frank supportive discussion will often move them to seek the help they need.

Guilt

Guilt refers to a feeling of responsibility for something combined with the belief that it could or should have been handled differently. Defined in this way, guilt is common in dementia caregivers. In our research, guilt is more common in family members who care for someone with dementia than in family members who care for a person with another chronic illness. This research also found that guilt declined over time in the caregivers of persons with dementia. Why should guilt be more common in caregivers of the demented? We can only speculate, but several explanations seem plausible. Dementia, unlike most other chronic illnesses, ultimately impairs the ill person's capacity to understand current circumstances and plan for the future. This is not true in every person with dementia, but the majority, particularly those with Alzheimer disease, are unaware that their memory is deteriorating and that they are less able to care for themselves. This combination of a lack of awareness and impaired decision making capacity puts family members in a very difficult position—it forces them to make difficult decisions for another adult. Frequently, these decisions involve choices that neither the ill person nor the family would have made before the dementing illness. Even worse, they are often actions that the ill individual dislikes—for example, being told he cannot drive or go out for a walk on his own; having his checkbook taken away; being taken to a daycare center; being admitted to a nursing home; or, being brought to a doctor to have his memory evaluated. Each of these actions may be necessary and is being done for the benefit of the ill person. Nonetheless, many families feel guilty that they have to decide such important matters for another adult, even when they know that they are doing "the right thing." The fact that the ill person may disagree or is often unable to say "Thank you" makes these actions even more difficult and more guilt provoking.

Some writers and thinkers have referred to this act of making decisions for a parent or spouse as "role reversal." We agree with Elaine Brody that this phrase is inaccurate because it misses the dilemma experienced by the caregiver. It is more accurate to say that many family members are *conflicted* about the changes forced upon their relationship with the ill person. The child who has to tell a parent what to do, the husband who can no longer rely on his wife's advice about children or grandchildren, and the wife who must tell her husband that he can no longer drive—all face the awareness they must act differently toward the ill person than they did prior to the dementia. It seems incorrect to say that the relationship (parent, child, spouse, lover) has reversed since the long-term emotional bond is still present. What *has* changed is that the healthy person must act differently toward the ill person. This can require a change in some aspects of role (decisionmaker, planner, food preparer), but there is almost never a complete reversal of the prior relationships. Whatever one calls it, though, this *change* in role is a common source of guilt.

Guilt can also arise because caregivers feel they have failed to uphold a longstanding belief or desire. Most cultures share the belief that it is the family's duty to care for a disabled family member. This value is sometimes transformed into a belief that it is *wrong* to seek help from others. As a result, some caregivers perceive that asking for help from family, friends, or professionals, placing a loved one in a long-term-care facility, or using others to bathe, dress, and feed a loved one means that they have failed. This feeling is made worse if the ill person believes that help is unnecessary and resists it. Since Alzheimer disease causes an inability to appreciate the need, unwarranted guilt in the caregiver commonly follows.

Fatigue

Some patients need to be dressed, fed, and bathed. Others develop balance problems and need help walking. Some become unable to walk. Since most caregivers have multiple responsibilities that go beyond physical care and because many are older and frail themselves, these requirements can become overwhelming. The fatigue that results worsens demoralization and robs the caregiver of the ability to derive enjoyment from other activities. Fatigue may even become a health problem for the caregiver. Therefore, tiredness, low energy, and poor sleep are indications that caregivers need more help than they are currently receiving.

THE NON-FAMILY CAREGIVER

In the United States 30%–50% of dementia patients receive care from nonfamily caregivers. Some are aides or nursing assistants hired directly by the family to care for someone in a home setting. Others work for home-health agencies, assisted living settings, retirement communities, hospitals, or nursing homes. Most are aides, practical nurses, licensed nurses, or geriatric assistants. Many have little or no training in the care of persons with dementia.

The small amount of research that has examined these non-family caregivers suggests that they have the same emotional responses to caregiving as do family caregivers, even though they tend to work in shifts and usually do not have long-term personal involvement with the patient. Being attentive to one's emotional needs and knowing how to approach the problems that arise in care are as important for the professional caregiver as they are for the family caregiver.

HELPING THE FAMILY AND PROFESSIONAL
CARE PROVIDER

Even though almost all the dementias are currently irreversible, a great deal of help is available. This is an important message for caregivers and the public at large because the emphasis placed on cure and prevention by the U.S. health system implies that chronic, progressive diseases like the dementias are unimportant and untreatable.

It is important to realize, nevertheless, that there are limits to what can be done to treat dementia. Some symptoms don't respond to the treatments we try and others improve only partially. Furthermore, the emotional, physical, social, and financial resources of patients, families, and society are limited. In spite of these challenges, the principles outlined in Chapter 5 are powerful and compelling reasons to provide treatment and to include the caregivers/families as a focus of care.

Since not all caregivers need professional help, should we wait until people become distressed and overwhelmed before we offer them help? The answer to this is clearly, "no." Research is beginning to help us identify which caregivers are at high risk of having a difficult time with caregiving and for whom preventive interventions might be especially helpful. One study has shown that a series of meetings with caregivers in the weeks following diagnosis results in long term mood improvement in the care provider and a delay in nursing home placement.

Research also shows that caregivers who feel supported by their spiritual or religious beliefs are less likely to be distressed and less likely to become demoralized over time. These studies also find that being able to find spiritual meaning in difficult situations is more important than actual attendance at religious services. This may be true because many caregivers who are unable to attend formal services because of the dementia are still able to find meaning in this difficult, adverse situation.

One unexpected finding from research is that greater severity of dementia does not increase the caregiver's need for emotional support or help. Perhaps this is why an intervention early in the course of dementia can have benefits years later. Most studies have also shown that it is the caregiver's *perception* of whether a particular issue is a problem rather than the objectively measured severity of a specific symptom that determines whether the caregiver needs help. As stated previously, there is not a direct relationship between disease severity and burden. Professionals must therefore directly ask about caregivers' perception of stress.

The importance of caregivers' perceptions of the situation and of their ability to give meaning to the situation demonstrates that each caregiver must be treated as an individual. Caregivers' innate psychological resources, in combination with their interpersonal, intellectual, and financial resources, are major determinants of how distressed they are likely to become. It is the professional's job to elicit information about each of these, to integrate this with the assessment of the patient's needs, and to recommend a treatment plan that is most likely to help that family.

Regular reassessment, ideally every 4–6 months, is helpful. This can help the clinician develop a long term relationship with the caregiver and can make it easier for the caregiver to ask for help when needed. Reassessment should also be triggered by major changes in the patient's clinical status, the caregiver's status, or caregiving circumstances (e.g., a housing move).

General Approaches

Although we emphasize the unique aspects of each caregiver's situation, there are some approaches that we use frequently.

Repeat information. Families and patients receive a great deal of new information from clinicians, friends, and the media, much of it in the form of bad news. It is not surprising, therefore, that they do not absorb everything they are being told. For this reason, clinicians should try to identify when they "haven't gotten through." Specific, direct information is most likely to be understood but repetition is often necessary. Providing written information in the form of brochures and books can complement a discussion and reinforce what is being said. Clinicians should ask if there are questions but keep in mind that many people are intimidated by professionals and do not ask their questions or acknowledge that they don't understand. Therefore, anticipating common questions ("A lot of people ask about . . .") and offering to repeat things are strategies that make it easier to provide the repetition some people need.

Give caregivers a feeling of hope. The demonstration that things can be done to improve a situation is important. Clinicians who identify the symptoms that may improve and acknowledge that some cannot generate realistic optimism and help caregivers begin to accept the parts of the illness that cannot be changed.

Listen for myths and misunderstandings. Society, individuals, and professionals share many incorrect ideas about the dementias. The clinician should listen for these and attempt to correct them if they arise. For example, some caregivers worry that the ill person will "go crazy." This is such a broad phrase that it has very little meaning, but usually it reflects the concern that the ill person will become violent or aggressive, that behavior will be unpredictable, and that nothing can be done to help. It is important to point out that agitated behavior does occur, but only in a minority of individuals. More importantly, most patients who develop such symptoms can be helped with available treatments. Some people believe that inactivity, lifestyle, diet, or particular behaviors can cause Alzheimer disease. There is no evidence that these are significant risk factors. Another common concern of care-providers is that they waited too long to bring the patient to medical attention. Exploration of this issue usually reveals that earlier diagnosis would not have made a significant difference to the patient or family.

Help the caregiver recognize that frequent distress in the patient is a sign that changes are necessary. Patients with dementia usually signal when something is beyond their ability even if they cannot say so. Indicators that patients are overwhelmed include frequent frustration, catastrophic reactions, and repeated resistance to certain tasks. These behaviors suggest that changes are needed in the environment, in the caregiver's approach, or both.

Encourage caregivers to use available resources. No single clinician can provide all the necessary legal, financial, medical, and resource information. The evaluating clinician should refer patients and families to a social worker, agency on aging, family support organization such as the Alzheimer's Association, or family community resources when issues arise about which they do not have expertise. Some families will have a family lawyer who can be consulted, but they may need advice from an expert in family law or geriatric law. Referral to a social worker, family services agency, financial planner, or geriatric care specialists can provide needed information. Families often resist such referrals, particularly when the symptoms of dementia are mild. It may be helpful to point out that an early awareness of available resources can delay or prevent problems from arising later.

Organize a family meeting. A meeting of family members, both those who are directly involved in caregiving and those who aren't, can accomplish several goals. It is common for those not directly involved in care to underestimate the stress of caregivers. The meeting allows for all involved to hear of the diagnosis and of current and future needs of the patient and primary caregivers. Often primary caregivers are reluctant to directly ask for help. The leader of the meeting can facilitate enlisting the help of others.

Listen for misdirected anger. Anger can be generated by many issues: the disease, the ill person who does something "wrong," family members who do not help more, professionals who do not make the proper diagnosis or are not being supportive enough, or society for not providing needed resources.

However, anger can be misdirected. A caregiver may be frustrated by one thing but end up expressing it toward something or someone else. This happens in many situations in life. A person may be frustrated at work or be disappointed in a relationship with another person and yet explode later at someone who has nothing to do with the disappointment. Among caregivers, anger at the disease, their situation or other problems might manifest itself as anger toward the ill person or other care providers.

Sometimes it is neither possible nor appropriate to express anger directly at its source. If the anger arises from an action of the patient, it is usually not appropriate to express the upset directly to the ill person since he or she cannot respond appropriately. In this instance, it is helpful to have other "outlets." It is often a relief just to express the anger in words to another person. Many people find that talking to a close friend or relative (a listening ear), participating in a support group, and keeping a journal are healthier ways of letting out anger. Persistent, angry feelings are usually an indicator that a person needs time away from caregiving or at least time away from a specific individual or situation. If anger persists after several attempts to correct misperceptions and redirect it, referral to a counselor or support group should be considered.

Provide caregivers with a nonjudgmental setting in which they can express feelings. Some caregivers are frightened or overwhelmed by their feelings of guilt, demoralization, or anger. It is usually helpful to be able to express these feelings openly. A supportive listening ear can help caregivers understand that their feelings are common among caregivers and do not make them a bad or uncaring person. Talking openly about feelings can provide relief in itself and may help caregivers think about *why* they are distressed. For example, some caregivers have not considered the fact that they are losing or have lost a loved one. Being able to discover a cause for feelings is helpful to many individuals.

Be available in a crisis. It should be anticipated that the patient's condition may progress and that crises will occur over time. Assuring caregivers of the availability of the clinical team can inspire great confidence. Such contact in the event of sudden changes in behavior also allows for appropriate triage, evaluation, and treatment.

Underlying Principles of Intervening with Caregivers

Several approaches underlie good caregiver support: education, problem solving, long-range planning, and addressing the emotional needs of caregivers. Each of these is combined in a prescription that may constantly change but which works best when all elements are present. For simplicity, they must be discussed separately. Professionals who provide care are like symphony conductors, knowing when to bring in and emphasize one or two elements but also knowing that the balance among these approaches is what makes the overall care work best.

Table 7.1 contains a list of interventions which must be considered for all caregivers, family, and professionals. The italicized items refer to interventions which might not be necessary for all caregivers.

Education. Well-informed caregivers are best equipped to address the problems that dementia presents. How much education caregivers need depends on their role in the caregiving situation, their ability to learn about a very complex situation, and their interest. Educational needs also vary over time because most dementias are progressive. Furthermore, caregivers' ability to comprehend, learn, and accept information may change over time. Most can absorb only so much information in one hearing, and their ability to learn may be affected by their emotional state.

People learn by different methods. Some learn best by listening, others by reading, and most by repetition. Written material is helpful for many people, and several advocacy organizations, including the Alzheimer's Association and the Brain Injury Association, provide excellent pamphlets on specific topics.

We believe that being informed about medical facts provides a sense of mastery because the problems of the individual ill person are placed into a framework that explains many aspects of the patient's presentation. However, we do not believe that a general understanding of the illness will explain all or even most of a person's problems. Helping caregivers identify which of the patient's symptoms arise from the brain injury and which likely have other causes is an important goal of the education process.

Teaching problem-solving skills. Patients with dementia develop many problems that neither they nor their caregivers have faced previously. We find that common sense problem solving is frequently effective. Even when solutions are only partially successful in resolving a problem, they can provide tremendous support to the ill person and the care provider. One of the benefits of focusing on common sense problem solving is that most individuals are able to learn the principles and use

Table 7.1. Caregiving Interventions

Education
  Dementia
    Cognitive impairments
    Functional impairments
    *Non-cognitive symptoms
  Diagnosis
  Prognosis
  Treatments (Chapters 6, 7, 8, 9, 10)
    Cognitive enhancing medications (Chapter 10)
    *Noncognitive symptoms (Chapter 8)
    Support of Patient (Chapter 6)
  Medications (Chapter10)
  Dispelling myths
  *Genetics
  Keeping up to date
  Research

Long-Range Planning
  Caregivers and responsibilities
  Resources and how to get them
  Residence plans and placement
  Late stage care (Chapter 11)

Decision Making and Advance Directives (Chapter 12)

*Resolving Family Conflict

*Coaching on How to Approach the Patient (Chapter 7)

*Problem-Solving Skills

*Legal–Financial Issues

Respite

*Individual Assessment and Treatment

*Attending to Personal Needs

Emotional Support
  Regular meetings and professional teams
  Availability
  *Support groups
  *Advocacy groups

*Interventions which might not be necessary with all caregivers.

them to address new problems when they arise. The problem-solving approaches that we advocate are emphasized in Chapters 9 and 10.

Addressing Specific Problems

Coaching how to approach the patient. Dementia usually changes the way people relate to each other. Some caregivers, family members, friends, and acquaintances have difficulty recognizing this and benefit from direct instruction about how to approach a person with dementia. There are emotional aspects of this issue which are dealt with in the next section. For many caregivers, knowing that it is the disease that is changing the person's behavior rather than the person doing something on purpose provides the insight through which they can change their approach. Some caregivers benefit by observing a clinician interact with the ill person and then meeting separately with the clinician to discuss how to approach the person. Occasionally, the clinician will need to demonstrate how particular actions of the caregiver distress or agitate the patient and how a change in approach can alter the undesirable interactions.

Long range planning. Caregiving for a person with dementia is a long-term affair. When the diagnosis is first made, some caregivers will be surprised that there is a problem. As the disease progresses, dementia forces role changes upon both the caregiver and the patient. Even if the dementia remains stable, there are changes in environment, family makeup, and medical status that require adaptation.

Long-range-planning issues include financial resources, legal needs (wills, powers of attorney) possible change in residence, and end of life decisions. While these issues may not arise for months or years, preliminary discussions are almost always beneficial. If they occur early in the course of the illness, the patient may be able to participate. However, it is impossible to anticipate all needs and attitude changes, so patients and families should be counseled to expect some planned choices to change in the future. Caregivers can be helped greatly by knowing the clinical team will assist with issues as they arise.

Respite: helping the caregiver accept outside help. In our opinion, time away from caregiving is a universal need of caregivers. It is often useful for the professional to point out early in the course of treatment that respite is necessary for all caregivers. It is also important for the professional to point out to other family members that providing help to the primary caregiver and allowing her time away from the caregiving situation will benefit all involved, including the ill person.

Respite can include having another family member or good friend spend several hours with the ill person, hiring a person to clean the house, or having someone stay with the ill person while the family member goes out shopping or visiting friends. It is best done on a routine and predictable basis.

Professional respite resources are available in some communities. Therefore, clinicians who do not know what is available should refer the caregiver to a social service agency or a clinician (such as a social worker) who is knowledgeable about available social services in that area. Some facilities provide overnight respite.

Some patients resist having a "stranger" come into the house or resist going to a daycare or overnight respite center. This is less likely if these activities become a practice early in caregiving, particularly when the patient is able to understand why it is being done. Often, a patient's resistance reflects the ambivalence or reluctance of the caregiver. When this is the case, the clinician should discuss this directly with the care provider. If the patient continues to resist, we suggest that the caregiver say that the respite worker is there to help the caregiver. For example, the caregiver might say, "This person is here to help me," rather than saying help is necessary because of the illness.

Scheduled respite usually works best. It is sometimes necessary for the professional caregiver to contact other family members directly and emphasize the importance to the primary caregiver of respite care. Making this an issue for the whole family to decide rather than for one individual lessens the burden on the primary caregiver and spreads the care among several family members.

Substitute decision making (see also Chapter 12). Because dementia impairs the capacities that underlie thinking, most dementias eventually rob the patient of the ability to make decisions. At the beginning of the illness, however, many patients have intact decision-making capacities. In the slowly progressive dementias, decision-making capacity is lost in a gradual manner, so there is no single time when a person goes from having the capacity to losing it. The ability to make complex decisions becomes impaired first; the ability to make less crucial decisions is retained until later in the disease.

This gradual loss of decision-making capacity places several demands on the caregiver. Although it is desirable that patients make decisions when they can, it is difficult to know when the capacity to make a specific decision has been lost. This is especially problematic in Alzheimer disease, since most patients with Alzheimer disease are unable to appreciate that their capacity to decide has become diminished or lost. The result is that family members or the legally appointed representatives need to be on guard, especially when complex issues are involved, and sometimes must override a patient's wishes. Professional caregivers can help families decide which decisions the ill person can still make, which decisions the ill person is unable to make, and which decisions should be made mutually.

The caregivers' or guardians' emotional reactions may keep them from making decisions for an ill person. When this is the case, the professional should point out to family members or the guardian the emotional challenges they are facing. Clinicians can help the family member make the necessary decisions but should not impose their judgments on the family. It often takes time for family members or a guardian to consider the issues, and there is often no reason to rush to a decision. The clinician can sometimes help the process by identifying the benefits and drawbacks of various options.

Helping caregivers address their personal needs. Caregiving is a time consuming activity, and some caregivers do not attend to their own personal needs. Medical and dental appointments, hobbies, meeting with friends and family, and going on vacations are examples of activities that some caregivers need to be reminded to do. Caregivers ignore their own needs so frequently that we routinely raise the issue when we first evaluate patients with dementia. A common reason that caregivers don't attend to their own needs is the prevalent belief that they provide the best care for their loved ones and, therefore, cannot leave the person with friends, family, or paid caregivers. We believe it is important to address this issue directly and point out to caregivers that it will benefit both them and the ill person if they pay attention to everyone's needs. Guilt and demoralization frequently interfere with the caregivers' ability to get away and should be addressed if they are preventing caregivers from attending to personal needs. This is another example for the frequent need to offer both practical solutions and emotional support.

Providing emotional support. While many caregivers report feeling emotionally overwhelmed by the caregiving experience, not all caregivers do. Elsewhere we address the importance of supplying appropriate information about the individual patient, the disease, and available community resources. Many discouraged caregivers also benefit by having direct attention paid to their mood. Research studies demonstrate that the most effective caregivers' support groups are those that provide both emotional support and education but that providing emotional support alone will improve caregiver distress more than will providing education alone. Therefore, we recommend that caregivers who are emotionally distressed or overwhelmed be provided with both. This can be done in individual meetings with clinicians or in support groups. Many individuals benefit from both. We believe it is important for caregivers to have a setting available in which they can express their frustrations and negative emotions. We also believe it best if the individuals providing counseling and running groups are knowledgeable about dementia so that they can provide support.

We do not believe there is evidence that any one kind of counseling is more beneficial than any other, but this is a controversial area. What is important is that the emotional concerns of caregivers are addressed and that practical problem solving be offered when needed. Providing emotional support requires knowing about the caregiver's prior pattern of response to difficulties and having a thorough knowledge of the individual care provider's strength and limitations.

Support groups. Many caregivers benefit emotionally from support groups. However, we do not believe that support group attendance is necessary or desirable for all caregivers. As noted earlier, some caregivers are doing well and do not seem to need the support and information provided by a group. Others are uncomfortable in a group situation and are better helped if they can meet individually with a clinician, counselor, or social service worker. The ability to benefit from support groups is likely to depend upon cultural background since support groups have been very successful in the United States but less so in other countries.

Extensive research and clinical experience identifies what makes support groups successful. One important aspect is the establishment of an atmosphere in which participants share experiences with other individuals who have faced the same problems. Another is the provision of a setting in which negative feelings are understood and accepted. Support groups are particularly powerful in helping caregivers recognize that they are not alone in facing a difficult situation, that the emotional challenges which dementia has brought to bear on them are understandable, and that help is available to solve the practical problems and social challenges they face. Many caregivers find it easier to accept support and advice about symptom management and the need for respite from other caregivers who are or have been in the same situation.

Several issues about the composition and leadership of support groups have not been fully resolved. Many researchers believe that there needs to be an identified group leader, but some groups appear to run well without an identified leader. Also controversial is whether the group can be run by an untrained individual or is best led by someone who has been trained to run groups. We do not believe there is adequate scientific evidence to make a definitive recommendation about either issue, but our experience is that having one person in the group who is responsible—for including as many participants as possible, for calling on new or quiet members, for stopping a discussion if most attendees feel it is not beneficial, and for keeping time—results in groups that are rated as more effective. It sometimes take the skills of a trained group leader to provide this important guidance.

One question that arises frequently is whether it is useful to provide different groups for old and new caregivers. People who are attending their first group or who have a relative or friend who has recently been diagnosed often have many specific questions about Alzheimer disease or dementia which are not of interest to more experienced group members. Therefore, when practical, having a separate group for carers of persons who have been recently diagnosed is useful. Another reason for having separate groups is that the problems of patients with severe dementia may frighten or overwhelm the caregiver of someone whose loved one has recently been diagnosed. However, experienced caregivers provide information and emotional support that is very valuable, so we generally recommend not having too many specialized groups.

One common problem in groups is the tendency for one or two individuals to monopolize a group. These individuals often feel that they have a great deal to teach the others. A sensitive group leader can be helpful if this happens by directing the conversation to other issues and by involving other caregivers. The leader can also address this problem by gently reminding the person who is monopolizing the group that it is important to hear from others.

Some support groups work well because most important topics are brought up by group members. Often, however, it is helpful for the group leader to have specific discussion topics in mind before the group starts. The group leader may not need to raise them if the group is running well or if they come up spontaneously. However, there are important topics, such as feelings of frustration, depression, or demoralization, that may not be addressed unless raised by the group leader. This issue can be brought up by noting that caregivers experience a variety of emotions. Group leaders who feel comfortable discussing their own feelings can provide a model which other attendees may follow. A common and important type of problem the group leader may need to address is an unreasonable belief, idea, assumption, or demand on the part of one group member. For example, some caregivers place unreasonable expectations on themselves or other family members ("I'll never place my husband in a nursing home"). Others put off difficult decisions or have unrealistic expectations of treatments, therapies or institutions. Support groups can point these out and do so in a manner that is supportive. ("I did that too and now I realize it was a mistake," or "I felt the same way.")

The skilled group leader listens for common themes and makes sure that the group addresses them when they do arise. The power of support groups comes from the realization that many of the experiences of caregivers are shared by most group members. This can be a re-moralizing and renewing insight.

Resolving family conflicts. In one study, 56% of caregivers reported significant disagreement among family members. This is not surprising since many of the problems discussed in this book are difficult ones and affect various family members differently. The issues contributing to family discord include relationships prior to the development of dementia, the emotional resources of individual family members, the geographic proximity of caregivers (it is a common experience that children who live outside of town underestimate the severity of the dementia and the challenges faced by the caregiver), involvement of multiple families (when there have been prior marriages), and the current economic, cultural, social, and religious values of individual family members.

The primary goal of resolving family conflicts in the context of dementia is to help the family provide the environment which will be best for the ill person and for family members. Therefore, it is useful to distinguish between conflicts which predate the dementia and those which have emerged because of the dementia. Even though these distinctions are complex and often difficult to make, they are important. It is often helpful to make this distinction explicit to family members. Focusing on current problems keeps the emphasis on trying to solve problems directly relevant to the dementia. Ideally, all involved family members should meet together, but this is not always possible. It is important to begin by making sure that all family members have an adequate understanding of the disease and of the ill person's condition at that time. The clinician should help the family identify the nature of the disagreements and focus the discussion on solving these issues. It is important to be knowledgeable about prior and current relationships among family members since this often makes the current problems more understandable and provides guidance about resolving whatever conflicts exist.

It is important to identify the opinions of all attendees. Sometimes the clinician needs to be directive and make specific suggestions. It is usually better for family members to come up with solutions themselves. The long-term goal is to help the family develop problem-solving skills so that they can better address future difficulties. When longstanding problems are identified that predate the dementia, the clinician should suggest to the family that they seek other counseling.

What is in the patient's best interest may conflict with what is in the family members' best interest. This is a common source of conflict. Making this explicit can help family members weigh potential drawbacks and benefits and enable them to resolve challenging dilemmas.

Placement (see also Chapter 6). When a diagnosis of dementia is made, the course cannot be predicted with any certainty. Because many patients with dementia require more care than the family members can provide, we urge all family caregivers to avoid making promises to the ill person about long-term living arrangements. We also tell families that a wide variety of caregiving options are available and that they cannot know ahead of time which will be best for the ill person.

Long term care out of the home is frequently necessary in later stage dementia. The decision-making process is aided when financial, emotional, and practical issues are addressed directly, when information is provided about the range of realistic options, and when there is recognition that this is a major life decision that might take weeks or months. Long term care options include daycare, in-home respite by family and friends, in-home respite by paid professionals, brief out-of-home overnight respite in facilities that provide this service, assisted living, and nursing home placement. It is important for the professional to recognize that the use of long-term care does not constitute a failure and to convey this to the family.

Placement out of the home is appropriate when the patient's needs are greater than can be provided by the caregiver in the home setting. There is rarely a single reason for placement. Most commonly, a combination of functional decline and cognitive impairment makes it necessary. Unmodifiable behavioral disturbance is a frequent contributor as well. We believe the decision to place the ill person in long-term care depends upon the needs of the patient and the family. Among the effects of dementia on the family that need to be considered are adverse effects on children, the need of family members to work, and the constant emotional and physical burdens on the caregiver.

It is sometimes appropriate for clinicians to give direct recommendations about placement. Some caregivers need "permission" to place the patient in long-term care, especially if they are not aware of how severe the illness has become or have not recognized that placement would be best for the family.

We generally recommend that family members visit a variety of facilities and suggest they do so before a crisis arises. Since it is rare that any single facility is right for every patient and family, many elements need to be considered. In addition to the elements discussed already, financial resources, travel time to the facility, the physical environment, and the background interests of other residents are factors to consider.

In choosing a facility, families should ask staff about their training in and knowledge of the care of patients with dementia and inquire about the availability of expert consultants. It is especially important that an activity stimulation program be present on site and that any resident who is able to participate be encouraged to do so.

Once long term placement has occurred, families should monitor care and raise concerns about problems when they arise. They should also be encouraged to express positive feelings when these are appropriate.

Many dementias ultimately lead to death. Chapter 11 discusses the challenges raised by the physical care of late stage disease. Common ethical dilemmas that arise in late stage care include placement of feeding tubes and treatment of new-onset medical illnesses. (These are discussed in Chapter 12.) Families' and patients' wishes regarding these can be discussed in advance but we find that opinions and decisions often change over time and that families sometimes make different decisions when a problem actually rises.

Addressing questions about genetics. The role of genetics in Alzheimer disease and other dementias is an area of active research. Many questions are unanswered and the knowledge base is changing so rapidly that we try to avoid making generalizations. In our opinion, a discussion of the genetics of Alzheimer disease and other dementias is appropriate in some circumstances but it is helpful for the clinician to know current information about genetic risks and influences. At present, we do not recommend genetic testing for unaffected individuals, but this is an area of ongoing debate. Genetic testing is discussed in greater depth in Chapter 13.

ADVOCACY GROUPS

Advocacy groups have been important sources of information about heart disease, cancer, and many other illnesses for over 50 years. In the United States, advocacy groups focused on dementia have been in operation since the 1970s. The many services these groups provide include information about the disease, up to date reviews of research findings, and suggestions about management of day-to-day problems. Many local Alzheimer's Association chapters offer support groups and provide information about respite resources within their community.

Many advocacy groups are active politically and seek funding for research, medical services, and social services. An important role of these groups is advocating before legislative bodies for improved funding of research and care. We believe positive advocacy is an important task of these associations but do not think it is appropriate to advocate against other groups ("Disease A gets too much money—more of that should go to disease B").

8

Noncognitive Behavioral and Psychiatric Disorders

*I*mpairments in cognition are the defining characteristics of dementia. However, much of the debility that patients experience derives from the impairments in functioning and from the disturbed behaviors that accompany dementia. One major theme of this book is the idea that dementia can be treated and managed by systematically addressing these impairments. Chapters 8 and 9 present a systematic approach to the assessment and management of both impairment in functioning and disturbances of behavior in dementia patients. The primary assumption of this approach is that distinguishing among different problems guides the development of appropriate interventions and improves outcomes. We call this "the 4D approach." It is presented in Table 8.1.

This approach is grounded in several principles. First, the impairments seen in dementia have multiple causes that can be distinguished from one another. Second, identifying the sources or causes of an impairment can lead to treatment strategies that are effective and beneficial to both the ill person and the care-provider. Third, there is usually no one best treatment for any functional impairment or behavioral disturbance. As a result, discovering the most effective intervention is often a trial and error process.

As outlined on Table 8.1, the first step of the 4D approach is *define and describe*. The main goal of this step is to define the clinical problem as specifically as possible. This requires a careful assessment of the patient and the environment based on information derived from the history, discussion with caregivers, physical examination, and laboratory studies.

TABLE 8.1. Overview of "the 4D Approach" to Mental, Behavioral, and Functional Disturbances

Define and Describe
  Describe the phenomenology of the problem
  When, where, how, with whom, and after what does the problem arise?

Decode (What are the Contributing Causes?)
  Cognitive disorder (aphasia, apraxia, agnosia, amnesia, executive disturbance)
  Recognizable psychiatric disorder or syndrome
  Medical or neurologic illness, or medication
  Environment
  Caregiver approach

Devise a Treatment Plan
  Does the problem need to be treated? Why?
  Which of the contributing causes can be removed or modified?
  Are there empirical or anecdotal treatments that can be tried?
  Are there common sense treatments or interventions that can be tried?

Determine if the Treatment Works
  What is the expected outcome?
  What is the anticipated time course of treatment response?
  Who will do what, and by when?
  How will emergencies be addressed?
  What is the fallback plan?
  What untoward effects of treatment are expected and how will they be
    monitored?

In the second phase, *decode*, the potential contributing causes and precipitants are identified by systematically examining five areas. First, because all patients with dementia suffer from a cognitive disorder, the effects of the specific *cognitive impairments* associated with each patient's dementia must be assessed. The second area looks for the presence of recognizable *psychiatric disorders* such as depression or delusions that might be causing or contributing to the current clinical problem. The third area is *medical illness* and its symptoms. Medication side effects, urinary tract infections, upper respiratory infections, pain, visual impairment, hearing impairment, constipation, arthritis, dizziness, headaches, and the exacerbation of existing chronic conditions such as diabetes, heart disease, and stroke are common contributors to disability. The fourth area to consider in the decoding process is the *environment*. Is it too cold? Too noisy and stimulating? Is there enough structure? Finally, the approach of the caregivers needs to be reviewed. Do they have a good understanding of dementia? Do they approach the patient carefully? Does he or she rush the patient?

In the third phase, clinicians and caregivers *devise* a management plan that flows out of the decoding process by trying environmental, behavioral, and pharmacologic approaches. It should be clear why an intervention is being tried, what the goals are, and who will do what, in what sequence, where, when, and for how long.

The fourth D, *determine*, is as critical as any. It involves setting a goal that is realistic and achievable. Since it is common for the first intervention to fail or be only partly successful, it is important to know when it is time to stop an intervention and try something else. Some interventions fail because they have not been implemented consistently rather than because they were ineffective. Having a goal sometimes enables the practitioner to see that partial progress has been made and that persistence is in order.

Chapters 8 and 9 are structured around the four Ds. They discuss the more common clinical problems but certainly not all. The discussion in these chapters illustrates the approach to clinical problems and can be applied to many other problems in dementia care.

CATASTROPHIC REACTIONS

Define and Describe

The term *catastrophic reaction* refers to a sudden expression of negative emotion (such as crying or yelling) that is precipitated by an environmental event or a task failure. The phrase is useful because it expresses the idea that a person is behaving as if a catastrophe has happened even though the precipitant or stressor is a seemingly minor event. However, it is an awkward phrase because its meaning is not obvious and because it exaggerates what is occurring. Catastrophic reactions are associated with brain injury from any cause. These are common in individuals who have experienced head trauma and stroke and in persons with developmental disabilities.

Catastrophic reactions almost always begin suddenly. There is often a warning, however, so astute clinicians and caregivers can anticipate them. The premonitory signs vary from person to person. Common warning signs are motor restlessness, a facial expression of distress, increasing resistance to care, or a change in the tone of the person's voice. Sometimes a warning is observable but difficult to put into words. Catastrophic reactions often stop as abruptly as they begin.

The emotions expressed in a catastrophic reaction range from unhappiness and crying to anger and rage. Catastrophic reactions are often accompanied by heightened physical activity and sometimes by aggression. Several of the behavioral problems discussed in this chapter, including physical aggression, running away, intermittent yelling out, and crying, can be manifestations of catastrophic reactions.

The occurrence of frequent catastrophic reactions is a sign that the environment is overwhelming for the patient. It is important, though, not to conclude that the environment is "at fault." For example, catastrophic reactions can be precipitated by necessary activities such as bathing, feeding, or dressing. Sometimes a careful assessment and the patience to try several approaches during these activities may decrease the frequency or totally prevent the catastrophic reactions from occurring There are many instances, though, when the best that can be done is to decrease the severity and frequency of the catastrophic reaction by reducing exposure to precipitants.

Frequent catastrophic reactions may indicate that expectations are too high or that an activity that a patient was previously able to perform and enjoy is now overwhelming. The repeated occurrence of catastrophic reactions later in the day suggests that the person is fatigued and that a change in schedule is indicated.

Decode

Cognitive disorder. Catastrophic reactions can be precipitated by an inability to remember. An example is the patient who becomes frantic when a caregiver leaves the room. The inability to express needs or wants or to comprehend what is being said (aphasia) is also a frequent cause. An inability to perform an action that was previously easy to do (apraxia) is one of the most common causes of catastrophic reactions. Many of the problems that occur around dressing, bathing, or grooming are catastrophic reactions precipitated by apraxias. Since catastrophic reactions reflect a loss of usual control of emotional expression, it is likely that damage to the frontal lobes—which play a major role in emotional and behavioral inhibition, attention, and appreciation of social cues—contributes significantly to their occurrence and persistence. Catastrophic reactions also occur with injuries to limbic (also called "emotional") circuits deep within the temporal lobes.

Psychiatric disorder. Catastrophic reactions are common manifestations of depression, illusions, hallucinations, delusions, and mania in patients with dementia. Delirium can disinhibit emotional control so catastrophic reactions may signal the onset of a new medical illness.

Medical Disorder. Any medical disorder, ranging from an exacerbation of a chronic disorder problem to the development of a new illness or medication toxicity can be a cause. Pain is a common precipitant. Sources of pain that should be considered include gum erosion, broken teeth, cavities, hip fracture, osteoarthritis, spine fractures, constipation, burning on urination, a beginning decubitus ulcer, a skin rash, and a cold. Therefore, a thorough physical examination is indicated whenever there is a change in frequency or the development of catastrophic reactions.

Environment. Environmental precipitants can range from a minor change in routine to a change in residence. Loud noises, such as fire alarms, construction, television, and overhead paging, can trigger catastrophic reactions. Common causes in long term care facilities include loud staff meetings, the calling out or yelling of other residents, a noisy dining room, or overcrowding.

Caregiver. Caregivers who rush patients, who insist that they do activities they can no longer do, or who make critical statements or speak too rapidly or too loudly can provoke catastrophic reactions. Touching or moving close to patients without having gained their attention is another common precipitant. It is important to avoid making caregivers feel guilty when catastrophic reactions occur; rather, one should help them to recognize their role in causing such reactions and to use this recognition to diminish the frequency of occurrence.

Devise

Identifying situations likely to precipitate catastrophic reactions leads to a care plan that seeks to lessen the frequency of the precipitants and subsequently of the catastrophic reactions themselves. If *certain individuals* are present when catastrophic reactions occur it is important for them to assess what they are doing and how they are doing it when the reaction occurs. If catastrophic reactions occur at *certain times* of the day, an attempt should be made to perform potential precipitating activities at other times. For example, if most catastrophic reactions occur later in the day, it is best to schedule doctor's appointments, trips, or visits in the morning.

Catastrophic reactions often occur in *certain places,* such as the bathroom. This is probably because most adults are used to performing bathroom functions in private, but the small size of bathrooms may also contribute. Apraxias that cause an inability to toilet, brush teeth, or bathe are frequent precipitants and are examples of causes that cannot be avoided. We recommend decreasing the frequency of bathing if this is a precipitant.

Understanding that task failure is a common precipitant of the catastrophic reaction can lead to innovative ways of preventing task failures. For example, if a person is no longer able to use a knife to cut food, the food can be cut in the kitchen by others. If trouble using buttons is a precipitant, the provision of clothing that does not require buttons or zippers—for example, pullover shirts or Velcro fasteners—might decrease frustration and lessen the frequency of catastrophic reactions.

When catastrophic reactions are just beginning, several steps can be taken to stop them or lessen their severity. First, individuals around the person should remain calm. Second, care-providers should make it clear, in a supportive, firm way, that they are in control. Statements that explain what is happening and at the same time provide reassurance are an effective way of doing this. For example, saying, "Don't worry Bill, I can help with that. It's not so bad. We can finish this together," demonstrates the recognition that they are upset, shows that you will help them, and makes it clear that control of the situation is not lost.

Distraction is an important tool in defusing a catastrophic reaction. If the precipitating stressor can be removed, the catastrophic reaction may be avoided, stopped, or diminished. Often the care-provider is able to stop the dressing, bathing, feeding, or other precipitating activity. However, there are times when it is best to quickly finish what is being done, all the while talking the patient through the activity. For example, "Ellen, we almost have your blouse on . . . Now straighten your arm . . . Let me pull it over your head . . . We're almost finished . . . I know this is hard for you, but I'm helping you and we will be done in a minute."

It is rarely necessary to physically restrain a person, and this should be avoided unless there is clear, imminent danger. For example, if a person is about to run out of a door into the street or is holding a sharp object, then physical restraint may be needed. However, distraction, talking the patient through, emotional support, and removal of the stressor are almost always more effective and less dangerous.

Catastrophic reactions are often frightening to caregivers and to others around the ill person. It is sometimes helpful, after the fact, to explain to the other individuals what happened and why it happened. It is important for the caregivers to appreciate that their own emotional state and those of others can precipitate or worsen catastrophic reactions.

The avoidance or diminution of catastrophic reactions embodies many of the principles discussed in Chapter 5. Early recognition may help prevent them. A careful assessment of who, what, when, and where may lead to common sense solutions. Several interventions are often necessary before a successful one is found, and catastrophic reactions cannot always be prevented or stopped. Since some precipitants cannot be avoided, understanding that catastrophic reactions arise from the brain injury and are precipitated by the environment is a crucial insight. However, failure to prevent them does not necessarily mean that the environment is unsupportive, inappropriate, or at fault.

Medications are prescribed when catastrophic reactions are frequent and dangerous and the patient has not responded to environmental approaches. We know of no study which specifically addresses the treatment of catastrophic reactions with medications. In our experience medications are only modestly effective in diminishing catastrophic reactions. Possible treatments are mood stabilizers, selective serotonin reuptake inhibitor (SSRI) antidepressants, or antipsychotics (see Chapter 10). In our practice, medication treatment is used only as a last resort. When catastrophic reactions are related to depression, mania, or delirium, appropriate treatment should lessen their occurrence.

Determine

Counting and charting the number of catastrophic reactions and rating their severity serves as the basis for determining if they are decreasing as a result of treatment. Successful strategies may fail in time. When catastrophic reactions increase in frequency, the process of assessment should begin anew, since this usually signals a change in cognitive, psychiatric, medical, or environmental status. If medications are prescribed, no more than 4 weeks should be allowed for a given agent or dose to show benefit.

UNCOOPERATIVENESS AND RESISTANCE TO CARE

Define and Describe

The definition of *uncooperativeness* varies in relation to where it is occurring, who the caregiver is, and the specific situation. The words *uncooperative* and *resistant* are unsatisfactory because they imply that the behavior is deliberate. In fact, resistance to care is often the result of multiple factors. Problem behaviors can be willful—patients might not want to do something they are fearful of—but most commonly they result from or are influenced by the impairments caused by the dementia. For example, patients who resist bathing may be unable to wash, recognize the caregiver, or recognize their own disabilities. Uncooperativeness might result from an apraxia or agnosia, or it might be understood as resulting from the distress of a person being undressed by someone perceived to be a stranger. In spite of the awkwardness of the term *uncooperativeness*, we will use it because it is a common complaint, identifies problem behaviors that can be further broken down and specified, and serves as a model for how rational interventions can be devised. We cannot define *uncooperativeness* or *resistance to care*, however, because each reflects the caregiver's perspective rather than a specific set of behaviors.

The threshold for defining a particular behavior as uncooperative often depends on the setting in which it occurs. In caregiving situations where there are no time pressures and caregivers can approach and reapproach a task, one avoids the problem of *restlessness*. In a nursing home where a nursing assistance is caring for eight to 10 residents, a behavior might be labeled as *uncooperative* if it delays the care process.

Uncooperativeness in a person still able to do the tasks in question should be distinguished from the inability to comply with requests because of an inability to hear or to comprehend. It is important to note whether the problem is intermittent or constant and whether it is associated with certain activities, events, or times of day.

Caregivers frequently conclude that resistance to care—for example, repeated undressing, grabbing the sink and refusing to enter the shower, calling out ("Help, call the police") or slapping at the caregiver or the air—is being done deliberately to frustrate them. This is certainly possible, but it is uncommon in our experience. Careful assessment almost always reveals that these difficult behaviors are a result of the person's defeats, the environment, and the emotional reactions of the ill person and the caregiver.

One aspect of dementia that contributes to the use of the terms *uncooperative* and *purposeful* is that behavior problems vary in frequency from day to day, from one caregiver to another, even from minute to minute. Often this inconsistency seems to make no sense. For example, a person may urinate in wastebaskets or on the floor but use the toilet when taken to the bathroom. Understanding that many behaviors result from the disease leads to strategies that can solve them and defuses the frustration and anger that many caregivers experience.

Cultural expectations and family values shape how a behavior is interpreted. Patients who pick up food with their hands can be viewed as difficult or rebellious ("Why can't he eat like an adult?") or embarrassing ("She always had such good manners"). Such a behavior may be embarrassing to care providers or may increase their workload, but it is rarely done to cause these feelings.

Other elements that influence how a behavior is interpreted include time pressures and the demands of competing responsibilities. For example, patients who take 45 minutes to dress may be late for breakfast or miss a doctor's appointment, so the slowness is identified as problematic. In this instance, the slowness is interfering with eating or going to doctors but the problem is the need to rush the patient.

Decode

Cognitive disorder. Amnesia can cause patients to forget they have already done something or that they are supposed to do something. They may not even remember that they have dentures ("I'm thirty-five, how could I have false teeth?"). Aphasia interferes with the ability to understand verbal or written instructions and is a common reason that requested actions, especially when complex, are not carried out. Apraxias are among the most common causes of uncooperative behavior. They can be difficult to recognize because a patient may be able to do part of an action or may be able to activate it intermittently. Apraxia should be suspected whenever patients perform part of an activity and then become upset or uncooperative, do an activity out of sequence (for example, try to pull on pants before their feet are in both pants legs or put a slip on top of a dress), or do an activity incorrectly (put toothpaste on a finger instead of on the toothbrush or put dirty dishes away in the cupboard). Apraxias can impair simple activities (getting into and out of a chair or car) as well complex ones (using a microwave, cooking a meal). Apraxias can be difficult to recognize in dementia because they begin subtly and progress slowly. As a result, they may only be noticed when the whole activity becomes impossible. Another reason for not recognizing an apraxia is that the caregiver has compensated for it without realizing it. This sometimes occurs to such an extent that the loss of ability is not recognized as a problem until the impairment is so severe that the patient can no longer do any elements of the task. Agnosias impair the ability to recognize caregivers, places, and objects (pills, clothing, food). They also impair the ability to recognize that one is ill and needs help. Each of these can contribute to the appearance of uncooperativeness.

Apathy causes a lack of motivation to engage in activities a person is capable of doing. It is a frequent source of frustration for the caregiver and often interpreted as intentional resistance. A grasp reflex may be misinterpreted as resistance if the patient grabs and holds onto bed rails, the care provider's clothing, or a hand and does not respond to a request or command to let go. The grasp reflex is activated by stimulating the inner surface of the hand (palm or fingers). It becomes stronger as someone or something pulls against it.

Psychiatric disorder. Depression is a common cause of apathy and withdrawal and may lead to resistance and negativism. In addition, depression can result in delusions that lead to resistant behavior. Examples of depressive delusions that interfere with function include the beliefs that a person cannot do things she is capable of doing, that she should not do something because she is bad, that someone is out to harm her, that activities are hopeless, or that something bad will happen if she does a

particular activity. Suspiciousness and delusions such as the belief that
the food is poisoned or that a stranger is in the home can lead to a refusal to eat, to take medications, to participate in activities, or to follow
instructions. Hallucinations may lead to behaviors such as fleeing a
house, calling the police, or refusing to go to bed because a stranger
is in the room or bed. Mania causes overactivity, pacing for hours,
refusal to eat, overconfidence, and irritability, all of which may lead to
uncooperativeness.

Medical disorder. Behaviors that result from pain, hearing deficits, visual
impairments, incontinence, and weakness may be misinterpreted as
uncooperativeness. Pain is particularly difficult to recognize in severely
ill, nonverbal patients. Withdrawal, guarding, or pushing others away
may be the only sign that a person is in pain. Akathisia may cause
patients to pace or move when they are asked or told not to. We are
aware of no specific medications that cause uncooperativeness but medications that impair cognition are likely to contribute to behavioral
resistance.

Environment. Environments that are overstimulating and noisy (for
example, television, paging systems) exacerbate the effects of cognitive
impairments and precipitate catastrophic reactions that are labeled "uncooperativeness." Common examples include busy dining rooms or activity areas with unfamiliar or confusing stimuli (for example, medication carts), poor contrast, and dim lighting. Soft, low chairs can
contribute to resistance because they are difficult to arise from.

Caregivers. Resistance to care is more likely when the caregiver is rushing, being demanding and critical, has unrealistic expectations, gives
complicated multistage commands, does not get the patient's attention
before starting an activity or making a request, and does not tailor the
approach to each individual's strength and limitation.

Devise

The principles that underlie the management of resistance to care and
uncooperativeness are those that run throughout the book: Identify the
problem as specifically as possible, determine potential causes and contributions, devise strategies that address the causes, and regularly re-
assess success and failure. Specifically, for each problem labeled by a
caregiver as uncooperativeness, it is helpful to ask: (1) *What* is the specific problem? (2) *Where* is it occurring and what other activities are
going on? (3) *When* is it occurring? For example, is there one time of
day that the problem is usually occurring? (4) With *whom* is the patient
uncooperative? Is it everyone or just some individuals?

When uncooperativeness is intermittent, it is important to review situations in which the patient was cooperative. If one caregiver is more successful than another, his/her approaches should be studied and replicated. It might be useful to have another person watch an activity when resistance is a routine occurrence. The observer may be able to identify subtle problems and recognize strategies which facilitate cooperation.

If resistance to care arises from amnesia, aphasia, apraxia, or agnosia, it is sometimes of help to tell patients what is about to happen and then talk them through each step, giving one instruction at a time. If simple language and repetition do not help, then nonverbal communication, such as touching the patient and helping guide the activity might be attempted. Sometimes a patient can imitate an activity, if the caregiver demonstrates it.

When apraxia is present, the task should be broken down into its most basic steps. Physical assistance should be provided. Instructions should be given one step at a time. ("Let's open the toothpaste tube . . . put it on the brush . . . put it in your mouth . . . move it back and forth, up and down.") Encouragement and praise should be provided frequently in a supportive tone. ("Good job . . . you're doing fine . . . we're almost done.") Imitating the task sometimes helps the patient get started and the activity then proceeds normally.

When it is clear that the patients are unable to perform part of a task, caregivers should do it for them. This works best if the patient is told that the caregiver will help them and then informs of each step as it is being done. Agnosias are best managed by caregivers' saying who they are, using a supportive tone of voice, keeping the task in the patients' line of sight, reminding them several times what is being done, and using both verbal (words and inflection) and nonverbal (touch, visual) cuing.

Making requests in the form of a statement rather than a question or order, saying, "it's time for your shower," rather than ordering a person to "take a shower" or asking, "do you want to take a shower?" may lessen resistance. Distraction sometimes helps. For example, a pleasant conversation, favorite food, or another person may momentarily take a resistant person's attention off a task; when started again several seconds or minutes later, the task may proceed without difficulty.

The identification of contributing psychiatric and medical conditions is an essential step in addressing uncooperativeness. Even if the condition cannot be immediately treated, caregivers may more easily empathize with the patient if they understand that the resistance is coming from a recognizable condition such as apathy, paralysis, depression, or pain.

Resistance to taking medication is common. Potential solutions include using liquid forms of medication, crushing pills and putting them in applesauce or a drink (if it is appropriate for the medicine to be dissolved), encouraging patients, "bribing" patients ("I'll take you to the sing-along as soon as you take this"), deceiving them ("Just try it this one time"—see Chapter 12 on Ethics), or giving medication only once a day at their best time of the day.

When patients become catastrophic during an activity, the activity should be stopped if possible and the patient should be distracted. If the task needs to be done it can be attempted later. The process of care should be reviewed in hopes of finding a way to avoid or minimize the recurrence of the catastrophic reaction or resistance.

Uncooperativeness due to a strong grasp reflex is best managed by very slowly removing the clothing, bed rail, or hand from the patient's grasp. Distraction may lead to a spontaneous release of the grasp. Giving the person something else to hold onto may enable the caregiver to complete whatever needs to be done. Offering an alternative to occupy the person's hands such as another article of clothing, can avoid a struggle. On occasion, the grasp is so strong or persistent that the finger needs to be pried off the object. This should be done gently and *very* slowly to avoid injury.

Medication should be considered when all other approaches have failed; when the patient, caregiver, or others are at risk of harm; or when a specific psychiatric symptom or syndrome that is known to respond to the medication is present. Even when medication is indicated, it is usually more effective to combine it with a behavioral–environmental approach. Antipsychotics, mood stabilizers, beta-blockers, and antidepressants, alone or in combination with each other, have shown some efficacy in our experience (Chapter 10).

Determine

Goals must be realistic. While some problems can be easily solved, others can only be partly improved or take months to solve. Failure of one strategy does not preclude success with another. It is important to set a specific time frame for the determination of success or failure of a particular strategy. If a strategy is partly effective, it may need to be modified. It is difficult to generalize about how many different strategies should be tried, but sometimes partial success is all that can be realistically accomplished. Occasionally, a problem gets better only with the passage of time, presumably because the disease process has progressed.

AGGRESSION/AGITATION

Define and Describe

Agitation and *aggression* are nonspecific terms used to describe a variety of disturbances. For some, *agitation* refers to an activated state in which patients are overactive and distressed. *Aggression* is defined as any act which does, or threatens to, lead to harm to any person or object. Most cases of aggression in dementia involve verbal aggression such as yelling, screaming, or threatening through body posture. Occasionally, patients with dementia engage in physical aggression such as hitting, pushing, or shoving. Some people limit the uses of the word *aggression* to instances in which harm is the intended outcome but this is not universally accepted as necessary. However, the words *agitation* and *aggression* are used so differently by people that we prefer to focus on the specific behavior, for example, "Hits when being bathed," whenever possible. A purely behavioral description is not always possible, however, and seemingly unprovoked aggression and agitation do occur. Most often, however, precipitant or provocation can be identified and a specific behavior can be focused upon. Aggression and agitation are serious problems in dementia because they can lead to injury, patient's distress, and distress in others.

When confronted with aggression, the clinician should describe the form the aggression takes, against whom it is directed, the context in which it occurs, and its consequences, such as injury. Time of day, frequency, and what the patient says also need to be determined.

Decode

Cognitive disorder. Patients with aphasia may become verbally or physically aggressive as part of a catastrophic reaction (see earlier in this chapter) when frustrated by being unable to express themselves or to understand something being said to them. Patients who have agnosia and do not recognize a person who is approaching them may become aggressive and strike out in self-defense. Executive disorder contributes to aggression by removing usual inhibitions of aggressive urges.

Psychiatric disorder. Aggression in dementia is a common consequence of delusions and hallucinations. Depression, mania, and sleep deprivation can also lead to agitation and aggression.

Medical disorder. New aggression in an otherwise stable patient is often due to delirium secondary to a new medical problem. Pain, constipation, and visual or hearing impairments predispose to the development of aggression, especially in patients with impaired communication. Steroids and dopamine agonist (for example, levo-dopa) medications may predispose to aggression.

Environment. Overstimulating environments, understimulating environments, and environments which lack adequate structure and activity are associated with aggression and agitation.

Caregiver. Being rushed, approached from behind, or spoken to harshley may provoke aggression. Conversely, caregivers who are supportive and attentive are less likely to provoke aggression even in stressful situations.

Devise

The identification of cognitive, psychiatric, medical, environmental, and caregiver precipitants dictates the general strategy for prevention. If aphasia, apraxia, agnosia, or executive dysfunction are contributing, caregivers should modify their approach to lessen the misperceptions caused by the symptom and the distress that they cause in the patient. The discussions under *Catastrophic Reactions* and *Agitation/Aggression* provide specific suggestions.

Since aggression and agitation are frequent manifestations of catastrophic reactions, the removal of a precipitant, distraction of the patient, and calmness on the part of the care provider can help defuse acute aggression and agitation. Avoidance of harm and protection of the frail are of primary importance. If there is a meaningful risk of harm, then the care provider must act to stop the behavior even if this means grabbing the patient. Many individuals with dementia are frail, so caution must be used in the rare event that force is used. Most often, though, the development of a catastrophic reaction can be stopped before physical aggression develops.

If a particular psychiatric symptom or syndrome such as delusions, depression, or mania is present, it should be treated. The same is true for an acute medical problem. Appropriate environmental modifications should be made. Caregivers should be educated about identifying precipitants of aggression in the patient they are caring for so that if the patient becomes irritable or otherwise upset, they can attempt to distract them or calm them so as to prevent an aggressive episode. Increasing staff or caregiver time with the patient, providing activities, and structuring the day also can reduce aggression and agitation. If aggression or agitation is occurring exclusively in the context of providing care, the professional and caregiver should review the process of care provision and modify it accordingly. Caregivers may need to learn how to protect themselves against violent patients by blocking arm swings, getting out of holds, or controlling hands.

If these approaches fail, management of aggression necessitates a consultation from a psychiatrist or other behavioral management expert. Occasionally, inpatient psychiatric care is appropriate because of the danger to others or the need for close supervision of medication trials.

If aggression is unprovoked or unexplained after careful evaluation, or if the danger to either the patient or another is significant, pharmacologic treatment is appropriate (Chapter 10). First-line agents have traditionally been the antipsychotics, such as risperidone, olanzapine, haloperidol, or thioridazine. Second-line agents include mood stabilizers (divalproex sodium, carbamazepine, and gabapentin), followed by SSRI antidepressants. Clinical trials have now demonstrated that antipsychotics and mood stabilizers lessen the occurrence of aggression. A trial comparing these two classes of drugs will be needed before a recommendation can be made regarding comparative efficacy. If the aggression seems driven by disinhibition, stimulants, levo-dopa, or amantadine might be used. If sexual aggression is present, progesterone or leuprolide might be used. Some clinicians believe that failure of the above alone or in combination can lead to consideration of electroconvulsive therapy (ECT), but its efficacy has not been adequately studied. Alternative treatments include beta-adrenergic-blockers (such as propranolol), the benzodiazepines, or combinations of medicines of different classes.

Determine

The primary goal of aggression management is complete resolution of aggression. If this is not possible, a secondary goal is the minimization of the aggression's consequences. The latter is especially appropriate when aggression occurs only during the provision of care.

Interventions to manage aggression require as much as a month to succeed. Pharmacologic treatment may require several medication trials in sequence and can take longer. At all times, it should be clear who is responsible for each intervention, how response to treatment is being assessed, and how long will be allowed before calling a given intervention a failure. On rare occasions, the process of controlling aggression can take months and require repeated hospitalizations.

WANDERING AND PACING

Define and Describe

Wandering is defined as physically moving about without a goal that is obvious to an observer. Individual patients often exhibit a pattern characteristic for them—for example, wandering aimlessly about while looking calm and content, wandering back and forth between two places, or wandering in a repetitive circular pattern around the perimeter of the nursing unit or a particular room.

Pacing, in contrast, is a driven, rapid walking. Pacing individuals often appear unable to stop or relax. The description of wandering and pacing behavior should include where, when, and how often the patient moves about.

On occasion, wandering or pacing presents risks to the patient or others. Escape is the most common reason an intervention is needed. If patients attempt to leave safe surroundings such as their own home or a nursing home, they must be redirected if they have lost some or all of the ability to recognize hazards such as stairwells, windows, or traffic or are at risk for falls and other injuries. Intervention is also appropriate for patients who repeatedly wander into other people's rooms in long-term care or assisted living. This is problematic because it is an intrusion into the privacy of another and can lead to physical or verbal retaliation against the wanderer.

However, individuals who simply wander around the perimeter of a room or up and down a hallway do not need to be stopped as long as they do not disrupt others. An occasional patient may pace to exhaustion or may be at risk for a fall or serious injury from wandering. Experts cannot agree on whether it is appropriate to restrain such patients in order to enforce periods of rest and nourishment or to prevent falls.

Decode

Cognitive disorder. Amnesia can prevent patients from learning where they are and why they are there. This can lead to their repeatedly looking for deceased relatives, home, and family, and wandering about to find them. Aphasia impairs the ability to ask for something or to understand what one has been told; it may result in patients wandering about looking for what they want (food, clothes, or people). Apraxia of gait can increase the risk of falls and self-injury and necessitate an intervention. Agnosic patients are unable to recognize familiar places and people. They may wander about as they look for something or someone familiar.

Psychiatric disorder. Mood disorder may result in variable activity over time. Depressed individuals are usually less mobile early in the day and more active in the afternoon and evening. Depression can cause early morning awakening or frequent awakenings, and these can lead to nighttime wandering. Causes also include hallucinations, illusions, and delusions. One patient of ours repeatedly heard a voice (an auditory hallucination) saying, "Your children are burning, your children are burning" and paced around the nursing home until she fell to the floor in exhaustion looking for them.

Medical disorders. Hunger, thirst, and the need to urinate are universal human states that may lead to wandering. The need to use the bathroom is suggested by patients' tugging at their clothing and looking anxious. Pain, even due to minor conditions such as a rash, can cause discomfort and lead to wandering. Common causes of pain include headaches, dental pain, sinus congestion, arthritis, constipation, and gynecological disorders. Wandering may be the first symptom of medical conditions such as urinary tract infection, urinary retention, hyperthyroidism, and delirium.

Akathisia due to antipsychotic medications causes restlessness and pacing. Patients with Parkinson disease and other basal ganglia disorders may develop akathisia due to their disease. The chorea of Huntington disease sometimes leads to a characteristic lurching walk that resembles pacing. Medications that cause stimulation may increase motor activity and stimulate pacing. These include thyroid replacement, drugs, stimulants, pseudoephedrine, and theophylline. Diuretics causing frequent urination may induce wandering. Excessive consumption of caffeine can lead to restlessness, pacing, and wandering.

Environment. Wandering may be a response to an overstimulating, noisy environment or a response to the yelling or calling out of others. Wandering at shift change in a nursing home may be cued by seeing the nursing staff leave either because it suggests it is time to go home from work or as the result of less observation by staff. Other visual clues that can suggest to patients that they try to leave are coats and hats, passing cars, or visitors leaving. Ironically, lack of stimulation can also induce wandering. For example, the person who is left alone may wander outside to look for someone.

Caregiver. Patients may wander in an effort to get away from caregiving which upsets them. A more common problem, however, is the caregiver who attempts to interrupt pacing or wandering and precipitates a catastrophic reaction or aggressive act.

Devise

Specific causes of wandering or pacing, such as akathisia or other medical or psychiatric disorders, should be treated appropriately. There should be a review of the patient's daily routines and response to activity and distractions. Caregivers should be educated about wandering and reminded of the hazards associated with trying to stop it. When possible, caregivers can walk along with the patient or provide adequate space for the behavior to occur.

If the wandering is an effort to communicate a feeling or need, caregivers should observe and recognize cues promptly; for example, caregivers should assure that appropriate food and drink are available throughout the day and not assume that patients can find food and water when they need them. Increasing scheduled activities is one of the best methods for decreasing wandering.

Unwanted cues should be kept out of sight. If overstimulation is contributing, noise and lighting should be decreased or the patient should be taken to a less busy environment. The patient might be sheltered in an area where they cannot observe the coming and going of staff. Small changes in environment such as moving to another corridor of a nursing home, to a new setting, can result in wandering about for a period of days or weeks, but the behavior often lessens over time.

The risks and benefits of wandering should be reviewed with caregivers. Windows should have stops so that they can only be opened 6 inches and doors should have locks which are out of the patient's sight—for example, a hook-and-eye lock at the very top or at the bottom of the door. Many nursing centers and adult daycare centers have outside wandering gardens for patients to have freedom of movement. Even with the best design, a patient can occasionally climb a fence and escape. Thus, patients must be supervised even when they are in seemingly secure areas.

Medications to reduce wandering are rarely beneficial and are best avoided. In rare instances amantadine, stimulants, SSRI antidepressants, and mood stabilizers have been helpful (Chapter 10). In addition, some data suggest that the cholinesterase inhibitors (such as donepezil may reduce wandering and pacing. Restraints are indicated for wandering only when the risk of harm is significant.

Determine

Most interventions to treat wandering, other than those cases where a cause might be identified and treated, aim at permitting the wandering to occur in a safe and contained manner. Necessary environmental modifications and caregiver education can usually be accomplished over a period of weeks. Safety modifications should be made as soon as possible, however. In cases where safety is compromised and physical restraint is considered, a careful review of the potential risks and benefits should be carried out with the family or guardian, and if implemented, reassessed regularly.

DELIRIUM

Define and Describe

The hallmark of delirium is an impairment in level of consciousness or sensorium. By this is meant distractibility, inattentiveness, disorientation, and an inability to sustain conversation or activity. Delirium is usually accompanied by a range of mental symptoms such as irritability, visual or auditory hallucinations, misperceptions, delusions, affective lability, depression, euphoria, and social withdrawal. Some patients are hypervigilant, active, and easily startled. Others are lethargic, withdrawn, or hard to arouse. Most cases of delirium begin suddenly and the symptoms usually resolve with treatment of the underlying cause. An acute general medical condition is the most common cause. The assessment and recognition of delirium can be complicated in patients with dementia because the impairment in cognition sometimes makes it difficult to determine whether or not sensorium is impaired. In cerebrovascular dementia and dementia of the Lewy body type, the cognitive impairment may wax and wane, giving the impression of fluctuations in sensorium.

Decode

Cognitive disorder. Memory impairment is common in delirium but aphasia, apraxia, agnosia, amnesia, and executive disorder are not. However, delirium will worsen these when they are already present. A waxing and waning level of alertness, the hallmark of delirium, is paralleled by fluctuations in cognitive performance.

Psychiatric disorder. Delirium can resemble any psychiatric disorder since almost any mental symptom can occur in delirium. Patients with major depression may be inattentive, functionally impaired, and confused and thus give the impression that they have delirium. The same may be true of patients with delusions or sleep disorders. Thus, while these conditions are unlikely to be causing or contributing to delirium, they need to be distinguished from it.

Medical disorder. Delirium is invariably caused by a condition or substance that is toxic to the brain as a whole. Thus, when delirium is diagnosed there must be an underlying physiologic cause and a detailed physical and laboratory examination must be initiated. The most common causes of delirium are medication toxicity and urinary tract infection. Dehydration, constipation, malnutrition and other infections are other common causes. Many cases of delirium are due to multiple concurrent physiologic disturbances, each one contributing to its development. Delirium typically resolves when the cause is corrected, but this may take days or weeks. Delirium should be distinguished from sleep apnea, in which daytime drowsiness is common because of awakenings. Snoring is a common symptom of sleep apnea.

Environment. Environmental influences rarely cause delirium but commonly influence its presentation. For example, dark or noisy environments increase the likelihood of hallucinations. In the past it was thought that environments lacking stimulation, activity, or windows cause delirium, but this does not appear to be the case.

Caregiver. Caregivers cannot cause delirium directly, but inattentive caregivers might allow an exposure to toxins or medications or risk dehydration by not encouraging adequate fluid intake. Caregivers who are not attuned to fluctuations in a patient's mental state or behavior might not recognize a delirium until it is more severe.

Devise

If the decode process identifies the medical problem(s) or medication(s) that is likely causing the delirium, the treatment is their modification or elimination. However, in up to half of cases of delirium, a definite cause is not found. In this situation, it is usually best to stop or to lower the dosage of as many medications as possible. Appropriate supportive care, good lighting, one-on-one attention, frequent reorientation, explanation of circumstances, and meticulous attention to the patient's personal care needs are essential aspects of the management of delirium. If delirium is persistent and accompanied by marked sleep disorder, the treatment of the sleep disorder (Chapter 9) with the use of bright light therapy or medication can provide symptomatic relief (Chapter 10).

Pharmacologic interventions are warranted if patients are persistently aggressive, engaging in dangerous behaviors, or suffering from delusions and hallucinations. Antipsychotic neuroleptic drugs are preferred, haloperidol being the most commonly used agent. Alternative agents include risperidone and other high potency antipsychotics such as trifluoperazine, fluphenazine and olanzapine (Chapter 10). Benzodiazepines (Chapter 10) should be used when sedation is the primary goal, but they may worsen the delirious state and further disinhibit the patient.

Determine

The primary goal of treating delirium is its resolution, which is accomplished by identifying and correcting the underlying cause. Improvement should occur within days or weeks but patients with dementia may require an even longer period of time to recover fully. This is an important issue in patients with dementia who undergo surgery, since postoperative delirium is common and prolongs the recovery time from the surgery.

When an underlying cause cannot be identified and the delirium becomes chronic (often in more advanced dementia), management is complicated. Patients can live for many months in a delirious state. They require intensive supportive medical care and rarely need physical restraints for protection. Medication is sometimes necessary to alleviate distressing symptoms. Chronic delirium signals a poor prognosis.

YELLING, CALLING OUT, AND SCREAMING

Define and Describe

Vocalizations such as yelling and constantly calling out are common in patients with moderate to severe dementia. These vocalizations include screaming, repeatedly calling a person's name, asking for help, or asking for something specific such as food. They also include repetitive sounds or syllables, moaning, or unintelligible noises.

Vocalizations may occur intermittently but often follow a diurnal pattern, usually worse in the afternoon or evening. Vocalizations are particularly disruptive in institutional settings, such as nursing homes, because they affect a large number of people. However, even when only one caregiver is involved they can produce significant distress in the care-provider. They may also be distressing to the person calling out, although many patients who call out repetitively say they are not distressed when asked. In long-term-care facilities vocalizations often trigger calling out by other residents, thus escalating the adverse effect on the millieu.

Vocalizations are of concern to care-providers because they indicate suffering in the patient. They also place the patient at risk of being hit or retaliated against by other residents in a nursing home. They also induce stress in caregivers and visitors to the home or nursing home. Distressing vocalizations can lead to the ill person's being removed from a nursing home area in which the majority of residents spend their time, such as a lounge or living room. This removal can lead to progressive social isolation. Vocalizations may also prevent patients from participating in stimulating or distracting activities. The vocalizations discussed here do not include verbal threats, which were dealt with in the section on aggression.

Decode

Identifying an underlying cause for yelling, calling out, or screaming is especially challenging. Information from direct care-providers, such as nursing assistants, is invaluable in identifying any potential cause(s).

Cognitive disorder. Repetitive syllables (called *palilalia*) are almost always seen in patients with severe aphasia. Patients with executive disturbances and frontal lobe damage will also often call out or scream repet-itively. Patients who are agnosic or aphasic may call out for help as they are trying to sort out what is going on in their environment.

Psychiatric disorder. Depressed mood is a common cause of calling out, as are fear, suspicion, paranoia, hallucinations, and delusions. In depres-sion, calling out may follow a diurnal pattern (usually worse in the af-ternoon or evening) and is accompanied by other evidence of depres-sion. If a patient appears fearful, delusions or hallucinations should be suspected.

Medical disorder. Physical discomfort, delirium, and pain are common causes of repetitive calling. Dental pain, unsuspected hip pain, shoulder or vertebral fractures, skin rashes, gastrointestinal (GI) distress, arthri-tis, constipation, and urinary tract infections are all common causes of discomfort, yelling, or calling out. Immobility itself may lead to discom-fort and calling out. Thirst and hunger result in calling out, especially in patients who are unable to ask for food or drink for whatever reason, including aphasia. Visual or hearing impairment can lead to calling out, either because of fear and isolation or because of the inability to communicate.

Environment. Noisy environments in which radio or television is con-stantly turned on may stimulate calling out. Environments with signifi-cant activity can be confusing or threatening to patients and a source of overstimulation. While the source of the distress may seem minor to caregivers, yelling may be the only means by which some patients can express their distress.

Caregiver. Caregiver contributions to calling out include understimula-tion; overstimulation; underappreciation of the patient's deficits, lead-ing to unrealistic expectations; or caregiver distress that adversely af-fects the patient.

Devise

If aphasia or miscommunication is contributing to calling out, it is im-portant that all caregivers be instructed on the best approach to the lan-guage disorder of the particular patient. Patients with severe aphasia or disinhibition may respond to calm, quiet, supportive environments and to nonverbal interventions such as touch or guidance with touch and gestures.

A patient may repeat statements such as asking for food or saying that something is about to occur (for example, "My mother is taking me home this afternoon"). He or she may respond to redirection or distraction by a caregiver who uses a confident and calm tone and manner. Sometimes it is necessary to lie to the patient to reduce his/her distress. (The ethical issue is discussed further in Chapter 12.)

Depression, delusions, and hallucinations respond best to treatments for those conditions. Fear and suspicion often respond to a supportive, nonthreatening environment with one-on-one attention. Most often these psychiatric symptoms require a combination of a supportive setting and pharmacotherapy.

Individuals who call out only in the late afternoon may be tired and may do better with a scheduled nap.

Whenever pain is suspected, a complete physical examination should be performed by a physician or a nurse practitioner. It is crucial that the skin be carefully assessed, that the teeth and gums be examined, and that the patient be palpated for potential bruises or fractures in the spine, hips, shoulders, and long bones. If delirium is present or possible, medications should be reviewed. On rare occasions, when the patient seems in pain but no source can be found, a trial of an analgesic medication (acetaminophen, a nonsteroidal agent, or possibly a narcotic) is worthwhile. If the calling out diminishes, a renewed search for a source of pain should be undertaken and medication continued as long as safe or until a specific cause is found.

If no cause can be identified and if the distress to the patient and other individuals is great or the behavior will lead to the patient's being forced to move, medication treatment (Chapter 10) may be used to help the patient inhibit the calling out or to produce sedation. SSRI antidepressants (such as sertraline, fluoxetine, or paroxetine), mood stabilizing anticonvulsants (such as divalproex sodium, carbamazepine, or gabapentin), antipsychotic agents (such as risperidone, olanzapine, or haloperidol), beta-adrenergic-blockers (such as propranolol), sedative-hypnotics (such as lorazepam), or other agents such as trazodone and doxepin have been reported to show efficacy in the literature and in anecdotal reports.

Determine

Yelling, calling out, and screaming are among the most challenging behavioral problems in dementia care. Management failure is common. A combination of treatment approaches is frequently necessary. Treatment goals include the reduction in the frequency or severity of calling out, a reduction in the disruptiveness of calling out to patients and others, and a reduction of risk that the patient faces as a result of calling out. Typically, treatment response requires several weeks to months and multiple attempts at different treatments.

MOOD PROBLEMS (DEPRESSION, ANXIETY, IRRITABILITY, MANIA)

Define and Describe

A variety of mood states are seen in patients with dementia. In *eu-thymia*, mood is generally normal for that person, fluctuating within its usual range and not persistently or markedly low or high. In *dys-thymia*, mood is sad, unhappy, blue, or bad. Sometimes crying, self-deprecation, and hopelessness are present. *Euphoria,* in contrast, refers to mood elevation. It may be accompanied by *irritability*, a mood state in which patients have a short fuse and react in a hostile or belligerent way to stimulation. *Labile* mood refers to frequent, rapid shifts of mood. Low or depressed mood should be distinguished from *apathy*, a state of diminished motivation, initiative, and activity that occurs in the absence of sadness.

Anxiety is a mood state in which individuals are fearful, tense, and physically aroused. It is often accompanied by rapid heartbeat, muscle tension, and feelings of panic. *Grief* is a mood state in which patients experience recurrent episodes of sadness (a "welling up") following a loss.

Variations in mood state occur as part of day-to-day living. These fluctuations are usually transient and linked to current circumstances. However, when mood becomes extreme, sustained, unresponsive to daily events, or markedly labile, it is often a source of distress or danger to the patient and others.

When a mood state is not only abnormal for the individual but is also accompanied by a recognizable set of signs and symptoms, a *mood syndrome* is diagnosed. Several mood syndromes are associated with dementia. In *major depressive episodes*, a diminished vital sense (trouble sleeping, trouble eating, trouble with energy, trouble with concentration), and a low self-attitude (self-deprecation, hopelessness, self-blame, diminished self-esteem, and feelings of being a burden to others) are seen.

The opposite of depression is the *hypomanic or manic syndrome*, a state of elevated euphoric or irritable mood, increased vital sense (less need for sleep, overtalkativeness, overactivity), and increased self-attitude (overconfidence, poor judgment, or grandiosity and grandiose delusions).

Panic disorder is characterized by recurrent episodes of the feeling that something terrible is about to happen (*panic attacks*). The patient often avoids situations in which these panic attacks occur. Panic attacks usually start suddenly and are accompanied by physiologic symptoms such as rapid heartbeat, an inability to catch one's breath, numbness, tingling, dizziness, and abdominal discomfort.

These mood syndromes are associated with a variety of adverse outcomes including mental suffering in the patients, deconditioning from the limited activity that accompanies depression, weight loss and dehydration from limited eating, exhaustion and falls from overactivity, victimization due to bad judgment, and suicide.

The abnormal mood states and mood syndrome associated with dementia can be difficult to diagnose. Patients may have trouble communicating their mood or knowing how sustained their mood change has been. Caregivers may not notice or be aware of changes in mood, even if they notice behaviors such as tearfulness, irritability, social withdrawal, or aggression that can signal a depression. Depression may not be recognized in persons with dementia because low mood is thought to be the logical result of becoming demented. Statements such as, "Well, wouldn't you be unhappy if you had Alzheimer disease?" or, "It makes sense that she's crying and not eating, she's unhappy living in a nursing home," indicate ignorance of the fact that abnormal mood states can improve if they are appropriately treated.

Decode

Cognitive disorder. Frustration resulting from the specific cognitive impairments (such as amnesia or agnosia) that occur with dementia can cause emotional upset even in patients who lack insight. This frustration is often manifested as a catastrophic reaction (see earlier in this Chapter) but may take the form of *transient* crying, sadness, or self-deprecating comments ("I'm useless"). Frustration should be differentiated from the persistent mood change seen in major or minor depression and from grief. The latter is seen in patients who forget that a loved one has died and become tearful when reminded of this loss. The tearfulness or grief occurs only in the context of being reminded of the death.

Psychiatric disorder. Patients with dementia who have a personal history or family history of mood disorder prior to developing dementia are at higher risk of developing depression. These usually represent recurrence of the pre-existing disorder or reactions of vulnerable people to the stress of dementia.

The presence of certain delusions referred to as *mood congruent delusions* should suggest to the clinician that major depression may be present. These include the conviction that a person is a burden to others, not worthy of being helped, that the situation is hopeless ("God should take me") or that food is poisoned.

Medical disorder. Medications (steroids, benzodiazepines, beta-blockers, reserpine), pancreatic and lung cancer, left frontal stroke or tumor, chronic lung disease (perhaps due to hypoxia), vitamin B_{12} deficiency, and endocrine disorders such as hypothyroidism and Cushing disease are associated with mood disorder. Pain, constipation, and urinary tract and other infections can cause persistent discomfort and present as abnormal mood states.

Environment. Changes in the environment, such as moving; or in daily routine; misinterpretations of sad television shows; or seeing objects from the past, such as pictures of deceased relatives, can induce sadness. Most patients adjust to major changes in their life or routine, but this can take weeks or months. Persistent adjustment difficulties may indicate the presence of a major depression.

Caregiver. The approach of the caregiver has a major effect on mood. Being critical, angry, unsupportive, or threatening can cause sadness, crying, or demoralization. Exposing patients to situations in which they are likely to fail increases the likelihood that they will become upset and tearful. There is also evidence that depression in the caregiver is associated with depression in the patient. It is not known which causes the other, but treatment of either the caregiver or patient can improve the mood of the other. It is important not to blame caregivers and to recognize and treat caregivers who are depressed, demoralized, or overwhelmed.

Devise

When an identifiable cause of the abnormal mood state or mood syndrome, such as a new medical problem, an environmental stressor, or a caregiver difficulty is identified, it should be corrected. Particular attention should be paid to whether the abnormal mood state or mood syndrome appears to be independent of the patient's circumstances and environmental stressors. If the depression is mild, intermittent or non-life threatening, environmental and behavioral interventions should be tried first. Increasing structure, activity, and predictability often benefits depressed, anxious, and irritable patients. Research has shown that identifying activities that the patient previously liked and increasing the time that the patient engages in them can improve mood in both the patient and caregiver. Activities the ill person can no longer do should be avoided.

When patients become acutely distressed, panic-stricken, irritable, or sad, reassurance should be provided. Distraction can decrease the amount of time spent in the abnormal mood state, but it is time and labor intensive because it requires one-on-one attention for long periods of time. When possible, patients with abnormal mood states should be enrolled in day programs since they provide both distraction and structure.

If there is an abnormal mood state or mood syndrome that is not responsive to the above or if the mood state clearly meets criteria for major depression, then pharmacologic treatments should be considered. The treatment of depression, mania, and irritability with medications and ECT is discussed in Chapter 10.

Interventions for mood disorder may increase the emotional, physical, or financial burdens on caregivers. These should be addressed to increase the likelihood of success.

Determine

The goal of treating an abnormal mood state or mood syndrome is complete resolution of the problem. This is achievable in the majority of cases but not always. Typically, environmental and psychosocial interventions require the involvement of the caregiver. Measuring success often requires determining if the caregiver is able to carry out the recommended care plan.

If medications are used, 6–8 weeks should be allowed for a response. If improvement does not occur, a change in dosage or type of medication should be considered. Electroconvulsive therapy (ECT) should be considered if the depression is severe or life threatening or several medications have failed.

SEEING THINGS, HEARING VOICES, HALLUCINATIONS, AND ILLUSIONS

Define and Describe

Hallucinations are sensory perceptions without stimuli. Hallucinations can occur in any of the five senses but visual and auditory hallucinations are most common in dementia. It is essential that hallucinations be distinguished from illusions. *Illusions* are misperceptions of sensory stimuli that are actually present. Illusions are also common in dementia. They differ from hallucinations in that an object is present but is incorrectly perceived. For example, reporting that a chair in a dimly lit room is a person is an illusion; seeing a person in a clearly lit room when there is no one there is an hallucination. The distinction is important because illusions can often be eliminated by environmental changes such as improved lighting or removing confusing objects, but hallucinations infrequently respond to such interventions. Hallucinations should be distinguished from delusions, which are false *beliefs*. Hallucinations and delusions sometimes occur together.

Patients with dementia who hallucinate commonly report seeing people in their home or hearing people talk to them. Illusions almost always occur in the visual modality and are more likely to occur in circumstances of partial sensory deprivation such as low lighting. Both hallucinations and illusions are more likely to occur in patients who have impairments in vision or hearing.

Decode

Cognitive disorder. Hallucinations and illusions become more common as cognitive impairment worsens, probably reflecting the fact that the brain damage is becoming more widespread. Cognitive state may also affect how the patient reacts to a hallucination. Individuals with more severe cognitive impairments, especially those who are unable to communicate their experiences, seem more likely to become explosive, aggressive, or catastrophic in response to a hallucination or an illusion. There are no specific associations between hallucinations and aphasia, agnosia, apraxia, or executive function disturbances.

Psychiatric disorder. Hallucinations and illusions are specific psychiatric symptoms. In addition to dementia, they are also seen in delirium, schizophrenia, major depression, mania, and alcohol or drug intoxication or withdrawal.

Medical disorder. Acute brain injury (for example, stroke), alcohol withdrawal, or seizures can precipitate auditory or visual hallucinations. Any metabolic infection or toxic disorder that causes delirium can induce hallucinations. Impairments in visual acuity or hearing are risk factors for developing hallucinations. Certain classes of drugs, especially benzodiazepines, anticholinergics, steroids, and dopamine agonists (levo-dopa and many others) are associated with hallucinations.

Environments. Environments that encourage sensory deprivation, such as poorly lighted rooms, may predispose to illusions and hallucinations. Conversely, settings that are very noisy—for example, those with loud air conditioners or noisy dining rooms—produce stimuli that can be misperceived as illusions.

Caregiver. Caregivers do not cause patients to have hallucinations or delusions, but their response can affect how the patient reacts to these distressing symptoms. Caregivers who are supportive; who attempt to distract the patient; and who are not challenging, scornful, or disdainful are more likely to help the patient avoid becoming markedly distressed or upset when they hallucinate.

Devise

If a specific psychiatric syndrome such as delirium, schizophrenia or mood disorder is present, it should be treated appropriately. Medications that might be causing hallucinations and delusions should be discontinued, if possible, or lowered in dose. Medical conditions such as urinary tract infection, pneumonia, and acute stroke should be considered and treated if present. If impaired vision or hearing is present it should be corrected as much as possible with glasses or hearing aids or by removing cataracts.

It is important to determine how the hallucination or illusion is affecting the patient. Some individuals find these experiences comforting. One of our patients, for example, had a hallucination of a loving mother talking to her. Often, however, hallucinations are frightening and cause patients to become aggressive or to try to get away.

If patients become upset in response to a hallucination, they should be comforted and calmed. The goal is to reduce distress rather than to remove the experience. Sometimes this is all that is needed whenever the patient becomes symptomatic. Reassurance and distraction often help. ("Bill, I know you're upset. Can you come over here and help me?")

It rarely helps to challenge the person ("I don't see anything. What are you talking about?"). Occasionally, it helps to acknowledge that the person is hallucinating ("I know you see the children but I don't"), but this approach often upsets the patient more. When possible, modifications to the environment should be made to increase ambient lighting, reduce the density of people around the patient, and reduce the sensory overstimulation associated with loud noises, running children, and television. These interventions are more likely to help diminish illusions than hallucinations.

When hallucinations are troubling to the patient and neither support nor simple environmental modifications relieve the distress, antipsychotic medication should be considered. Low doses of high-potency and "atypical" neuroleptics (such as risperidone, olanzapine, thiothixene, or haloperidol) are less likely to cause side effects. In our experience, while these drugs may diminish hallucinations, they almost never affect illusions. Chapter 10 discusses the use of these medications.

Determine

If a specific cause can be found and removed (for example, an eye problem, a medication, or a bladder infection), then abolishing the symptom is possible. However, for many patients, the primary goal is to reduce or minimize the distress caused by hallucinations and illusions.

Distraction, reassurance, and environmental modification are often effective almost immediately. If pharmacologic treatments are tried, response should occur within several weeks of starting the medication. Sometimes pharmacotherapy does not abolish the hallucinations but helps the patient by reducing distress. If neither occurs, the medication should be stopped. If the medication has benefitted the patient, then the need for continuing its prescription should be monitored every 2–3 months. After 3–6 months, particularly if the dementia appears to have progressed, the dosage should be reduced gradually and then discontinued if there is no recurrence of the hallucinations.

SUSPICIOUSNESS, PARANOIA, AND DELUSIONS

Define and Describe

Patients with dementia develop a range of false or unusual beliefs. They may insist that someone is stealing their belongings, that a spouse is unfaithful, or that food is being poisoned. Some patients are suspicious and misinterpret the motives of others as being directed against them. In some instances, these beliefs are fixed and patients can't be talked out of them, even with evidence to the contrary. Occasionally they will drive the patients to behave in predictable ways. For example, those who feel that they are being robbed may hide their belongings so that they are not stolen. Then they may discover that they can't find something that they have hidden and believe that others have stolen it. Those who feel persecuted may barricade themselves in their room. Those believing their spouse is unfaithful may become aggressive or even violent toward the spouse. In many instances, these false beliefs are benign and do not lead to distress in the patient. Indeed, in most cases, patients can be talked out of these beliefs or distracted from them through activity and structure.

In as many as 25%–30% of patients, these beliefs become persistent. These are referred to as *delusions*—that is, fixed, false, idiosyncratic (specific to that individual) beliefs. The identification of delusions is important because it indicates that the patient is experiencing a symptom of the dementing disease, it gives a name to a problem which may be very distressing to the caregiver, and it often implies an avenue for successful treatment.

Decode

Cognitive disorder. Many suspicious, paranoid, or untrue ideas and beliefs that patients develop can be linked directly to the cognitive disorder. For example, amnesia causes patients to forget where they place things and leads to the idea that someone has stolen their belongings.

Alternatively, agnosia causes an inability to recognize the environment and leads to the state in which they believe that they are not in their house or room when they are. Aphasia may lead patients to make statements that others misinterpret as bizarre or false. Finally, executive dysfunction can lead patients to be disinhibited, socially inappropriate, and to express what is on their mind before they have had a chance to think it through and form a belief or opinion.

Psychiatric Disorder. Delusions and other false beliefs can be part of a major depression, a manic episode, or delirium.

Medical disorder. Some medications, in particular steroids, levo-dopa, and H_2 blockers, have been associated with the development of delusions in the absence of delirium. Patients with dementia due to Parkinson disease and stroke are prone to developing delusions. Delusions can be a symptom of a delirium due to any medical problem.

Environment. Environmental contributions to delusions are uncommon, but a cluttered environment may increase the likelihood of misplacing things. An environment that is too loud or too stimulating may lead patients to misinterpret events and develop persecutory beliefs about things going on around them.

Caregiver. Caregivers who speak in half sentences or mutter or who are irritable and impatient may give the patient the impression that they are trying to hurt them. This can give rise to misinterpretations, false beliefs, or even delusions. Spouse caregivers who are often absent may unknowingly be contributing to the patient's belief of infidelity. Caregivers who do not offer reassurance when patients are confused may also unknowingly be contributing to the development of false beliefs and misinterpretations.

Devise

Some patients are comforted by false beliefs and aggressive efforts to stop them are not appropriate. If associations are made between distressing delusions and environmental or caregiver approaches, these should be corrected. If delusions or suspiciousness is occurring in the context of a depression, medical disorder, or medication, appropriate action should be taken. In the context of mania or depression, treatment of both the delusions and the mood syndrome should be pursued simultaneously.

When there is no obvious cause and the delusion is chronic, the decisions of whether and how to treat are based on the extent to which the delusion or suspiciousness is distressing to the patient or places someone at risk of being harmed. The extent to which the problem burdens the caregiver is a lesser consideration.

If the risk of harm to the patient or others is low, behavioral psychological interventions should be instituted first. Frequent scheduled activities, distraction, one-on-one attention, removing clutter from the environment, and periodic separation of the person who is the target of the suspicions and the patient can reduce the frequency of misinterpretation and the development of false beliefs.

If patients are clearly delusional, and the delusions are either distressing to patients or leading to behavior that is a threat to the patient or others, pharmacologic treatments should be considered. Randomized controlled trials show that antipsychotics decrease the severity of delusions. Antipsychotics can be chosen from any group as discussed in Chapter 10. However, agents such as risperidone, olanzapine, and haloperidol are preferred because of their lower side effect profile. Patients with dementia who are delusional are more prone to developing the extrapyramidal side effects of antipsychotics than comparably aged nondemented individuals. Therefore, caution should be exercised whenever they are prescribed and an attempt should be made to find the lowest effective dose.

Determine

If the misinterpretations, false beliefs, or delusions are not distressing or dangerous, a reasonable goal of treatment is to prevent them from causing distress or escalating into dangerous behavior. In cases where there is serious distress or dangerousness and treatment using medications is attempted, noticeable improvement should be observed within 4–6 weeks. If this does not occur, the medication dosage should be adjusted or a new medication should be tried.

SOCIAL WITHDRAWAL AND APATHY

Define and Describe

Apathy is a state characterized by lack of initiative and motivation and a lack of interest in activities previously enjoyed. Apathetic individuals are inactive and seem content doing little or nothing. When they participate or follow directions they do so slowly and after persistent encouragement. Apathy is often present early in the subcortical dementias. It arises late in the cortical dementias. *Social withdrawal* refers to the active avoidance of interaction with others. The apathetic person is almost never active while the socially withdrawn person may be active when alone. The apathetic individual may attend a day center and appear content to do nothing, while the socially withdrawn person is more likely to try to leave or participate only in solitary activities. Ironically, the apathetic person may readily accompany a caregiver to activities and sit quietly for hours.

Apathy is a problem because being active and productive is considered a sign of health. Therefore, families complain when a loved one is inactive. Apathy can lead to frustration and anger in caregivers because the ill person is unresponsive to maximal amounts of encouragement and stimulation and because caregivers often restrict their own activity to be with the patient. When apathetic patients do respond to stimulation, their activity stops as soon as the encouragement or stimulation stops.

Social withdrawal is problematic for caregivers because there is an element of active resistance. It too can lead caregivers to socially isolate themselves. The resistive behavior of the withdrawn person can be socially distressing for the caregiver if publicly displayed.

Apathy and social withdrawal are characterized by a normal level of consciousness and should be distinguished from the drowsy, inattentive state of delirium.

Decode

Cognitive disorder. Social withdrawal can result from cognitive impairment. Patients who are aware that they are unable to remember (amnesia), converse (aphasia), participate in an activity (apraxia), or recognize other people (agnosia) may actively avoid participation in activities or discussion with others because of the embarrassment.

Apathy is a defining feature of the frontal-subcortical dementias and of executive disturbance. It is often accompanied by other signs and symptoms of impaired executive function such as slowed thinking, inattentiveness, and difficulty with decision making. Families often describe such patients as "bumps on a log."

Psychiatric disorder. Withdrawal and apathy can be symptoms of major depressive disorder. Depressed patients often complain of being unable to participate, think, or move. They may feel unworthy, hopeless, useless, and responsible for the ills of the world. Depression is a common cause of apathy and withdrawal and should be considered whenever they are present.

Suspicious ideas and delusional beliefs, whatever their cause, can lead to social isolation. Individuals who barricade themselves in their room may be doing so in response to a delusion or hallucination or may be trying to escape from a verbally or physically threatening roommate.

Apathy and social withdrawal can be symptoms of schizophrenia, delirium, panic disorder, or agoraphobia (the fear of outdoor spaces).

Medical disorder. Acute and chronic hypoxia caused by pneumonia, chronic lung disease, and other respiratory disorders can cause withdrawal and apathy. Hearing and visual impairment can lead to social withdrawal. Certain cancers—for example, pancreatic cancer—can cause paraneoplastic syndromes that include apathy as a symptom. Hypothyroidism, Addison disease, anemia, chronic renal failure, hepatic encephalopathy, diseases of the basal ganglia (Parkinson disease and Huntington disease), and hydrocephalus can cause apathy. Sleep apnea can cause daytime drowsiness and sleeping that mimics social withdrawal and apathy. Medications that cause apathy include antipsychotics, anticholinergics, tricyclic antidepressants, barbiturates, benzodiazepines, long-acting cardiac antiarrhythmias, beta-blockers, and alcohol.

Environment. Overstimulating environments that place excessive demands on patients can lead to social withdrawal. Noise, crowds of people, easily misinterpreted objects like medication carts, and too many activities can be overwhelming. An example is the busy dining room in a nursing home. Noisy, threatening, or physically aggressive residents can cause social withdrawal. Very active small children may overwhelm some individuals. The noise from TV and radio may be misinterpreted or may frighten a person with dementia and lead to social isolation.

Conversely, environments that are insufficiently stimulating exaggerate an underlying tendency to be apathetic. Patients who are quiet and inactive may "fall through the cracks" because they are easy to manage and care for. This is an example of the environment preventing recognition of a potentially treatable problem or condition.

Caregivers. Caregivers who are too demanding or who understimulate patients can contribute to social withdrawal. An incorrect assessment of the patient's capacities may induce social withdrawal. For example, attributing a lack of response to a proposed activity in a patient to a lack of interest rather than to a lost ability (for example, an inability to read) prevents the caregiver from assessing inactivity and planning appropriate activities. Patients cared for by abusive, critical, and neglectful caregivers can become socially withdrawn.

Devise

Treatable causes of apathy and social withdrawal such as depression, cataracts, deafness, hypothyroidism, or medication intoxication should be ruled out before a purely environmental treatment is initiated. Even when a potential cause is found, the treatment should include both specific and environmental interventions. Education is crucial because it helps the caregiver understand the source of the problem and develop realistic expectations and plans.

The ideal approach provides the amount of environmental stimulation appropriate to the capabilities and prior interests of each individual. However, sometimes patients' prior interests, capabilities, or social status prevents caregivers from trying interventions that might benefit them. Tossing a ball may seem undignified for a person who was a banker but may provide pleasurable stimulation. Because most dementias are progressive, caregivers must continually modify the type and level of stimulation. If the patient becomes repeatedly frustrated when encouraged, the caregiver should stop. Caregivers need to be aware that frustration in patients can demoralize and discourage patients and worsen withdrawal.

Stimulation is a double-edged sword and needs to be adjusted to the tolerance of the individual. It is sometimes necessary to stop stimulating patients when they become distressed or do not respond or when the caregiver becomes distressed.

If environmental stimulation is unsuccessful and the lack of activity is harming the ill person, depriving them of pleasure or preventing a spouse from maintaining a social life, pharmacologic treatment should be considered. Unfortunately, benefit is uncommon. Drugs that increase brain dopamine or serotonin activity are theoretically beneficial. These include amantadine, the antidepressant medications bupropion and SSRIs, and the stimulants methylphenidate and dexadrine (Chapter 10). Recent data also suggest that augmentation of acetylcholine neurotransmission with donepezil and other cholinesterase inhibitors may reduce apathy (Chapter 10).

Determine

If apathy or social withdrawal is associated with a specific psychiatric syndrome, medical condition, or medication, treatment response may take weeks or months. Specific target responses include participating longer in an activity or participating in new activities. Some severely apathetic patients are active as long as they are stimulated but sink into inactivity the instant the stimulation stops. This can place overwhelming demands on caregivers, especially if they are the sole caregiver. Pharmacologic treatments improve apathy within several weeks when they work.

One frustrating element of *environmental activation* is that the patients often forget what they did. When asked, they may say they have done nothing all day when they have just completed 45 minutes of exercise. This may be misinterpreted as being ungrateful, or the caregiver may question the benefit, and yet the patient's enjoyment is obvious while engaged in the activity. Therefore, family members and staff should check with an involved staff person before concluding that a person has been inactive.

Unfortunately, attempts to reduce apathy and social withdrawal can induce distress. Apathetic patients are often content to be left alone and become frustrated, angry, and even explosive if pushed or encouraged. If attempts to improve apathy fail, caregivers should be reassured that it is very unlikely that stimulation will alter the course of the illness and more likely that excessive stimulation would adversely affect quality of life. When apathy is the object of treatment it is important to keep in mind whether the treatment is for the patient or the caregiver. If there is no evidence that the patient is benefitting from the treatment, it should be stopped.

RUMMAGING AND HOARDING

Define and Describe

Rummaging refers to the behavior looking through, touching and moving objects about. Persons who are rummaging appear to be looking for something yet may continue to look through drawers or purses for hours. There are many examples of rummaging, including repeatedly going through purses, wallets, or brief cases, continuously going through the mail, counting money over and over again, moving clothing about in drawers.

Hoarding refers to the collecting of objects. Often, the objects which are hoarded have little value. Bits of paper, packets of sugar, pieces of food, and odd items of clothing such as buttons or socks are commonly hoarded objects. In some instances, the person with dementia hoards currency, mail including bills and checks, identification cards, keys and other items of value. Once hoarded, or put away safely, the person will not remember where they were placed and the process of rummaging or looking for them begins anew.

Rummaging and hoarding are rarely problems for the patient unless limits are set on them. Checks or similar items of value can be misplaced and cause harm.

Decode

Cognitive disorder. Forgetful patients may constantly rummage through drawers in order to reassure themselves possessions are safe. Rummaging may also be related to agnosia. Such patients may not recognize their own possessions and constantly be looking for something they recognize as familiar. Rummaging through items in a purse or wallet can provide cues or reassurance to the person of who she is. Difficulty in understanding the routine of the day can result in persons hoarding food, unsure when the next meal is coming. Disorientation to place can result in persons packing suitcases believing they "won't be staying here." Dysfunction of the frontal lobes leading to perseveration or stimulus bound behavior can result in a person's picking up any object he sees and putting it in a "safe place" or, that is, hoarding it.

Psychiatric disorder. Persons who are suspicious may hoard possessions in order to hide them from persons they do not trust. Persons who are very anxious can attempt to relieve anxiety by constantly rummaging and hoarding. Mania can cause overactivity and apparently purposeless behavior.

Medical disorders. These are unlikely to contribute to this behavior, unless the patient is in pain, confused, or searching for a bathroom in which to void.

Environment. Cues from the environment such as open closet doors or drawers with clothing hanging out can stimulate patients to explore them and move things about and put them in a place they perceive as safe. Environments in which all bedrooms appear the same, and are not personalized can lead the person with dementia to believe that someone else's belongings are his because he finds it in a room that looks like his while rummaging through the possessions of other persons. In such instances, possessions of others can be lost and the "rummager" a victim of retaliation by the person whose possessions were taken. Environments that are very cluttered may cue patients to move things about in an attempt to maintain order.

Caregiver. It is unlikely that caregiver approval contributes to this behavior, but many caregivers are upset by the behavior.

Devise

If rummaging and hoarding cause any minor disruptions such as an untidy room, drawer or closet, allowing access to a limited area by locking all drawers except one, or locking some closets but not others, may allow the behavior to continue without causing distress to the patient, who may derive benefit from it (lower anxiety, a pleasurable activity, something to do).

Hoarding that arises from amnesia, disinhibition, or perseveration is best managed by limiting access to valuable objects and providing stimulation and frequent redirection. Structured activity programs can diminish the frequency of rummaging and hoarding by occupying the time and attention of the patient.

Rummaging and hoarding that arise from suspiciousness, delusions, or mania, are best addressed through treating the primary psychiatric disorder (see other parts of this chapter).

Sometimes the best approach is to allow the behavior to happen but to minimize its impact by routinely checking for hoarded items such as food or possessions of others. Often the hoarders collect objects and put them in the same place. When this is the case, it may be better to check the room when they are involved elsewhere rather than to confront them.

Providing a box with familiar possessions such as photographs, knick knacks, keys, objects from prior jobs, hobbies or family activities can limit the behavior to manageable proportions. Similarly, giving the person an inactive check register or purse without money can occupy the person's time. Keep suitcases or other triggers out of view if possible. Replacing valuable jewelry with costume pieces can avoid the painful loss of an heirloom.

Making sure that the caregiver has copies of important identification cards, bank books, check registers, insurance policies and cards, photographs, and items of sentimental value can permit the patient to continue having the pleasure of continued use but avoid the harm and disappointment of loss. Establishing an inventory of important personal items can improve the chances that items will be returned to their owners.

Rummaging and hoarding can be more problematic in the long term care setting since it impinges on non-family members. This behavior can be poorly tolerated by the residents in long term care, whether they are cognitively intact or impaired. If this happens, then attempts to redirect the behavior or limit it to certain safe areas or objects is warranted.

Labeling clothing can allow for its proper return. In some facilities, bedrooms are locked during the day, limiting access to the possessions of others. Some people object to this solution, but if attentive activity and support are provided, then the patient benefits from the added stimulation.

Medications are rarely useful although efforts to reduce disinhibition may reduce the behaviors (see Chapter 10 for medications for disinhibition).

Determine

This is a difficult set of behaviors to stop, so a decrease in frequency, protection against the loss of valuable articles, or avoidance of victimization by others is a reasonable measure of success. Often the principal goal of treatment is to contain the rummaging and hoarding so as not to cause the patient distress, while keeping the caregiver satisfied.

Noncognitive Disorders of Functioning and Disturbances of Sleeping, Eating, and Sexuality

*T*his Chapter contains the detailed discussion of common problems and symptoms that patients with dementia face. The focus is on strategies to manage these symptoms. The 4D approach, as discussed in Chapter 8, is used. Disturbances of sleeping, eating, and sexuality, and non-cognitive disorders of functioning are covered here. Non-cognitive behavioral and psychiatric disorders were covered in Chapter 8. When reference is made to medication treatment, the reader should consult Chapter 10.

EATING PROBLEMS AND WEIGHT LOSS

Define and Describe

Problems with eating include: undereating, overeating, eating nonfoods, forgetting to chew and swallow, choking, food refusal, and weight loss. The average person with Alzheimer disease loses 2–4 pounds in weight per year; the average person over the age of 70 loses 1 pound per year on average. The reasons for this slight gradual weight loss are not well established but it is likely that many factors contribute.

The process of ingesting food in humans includes two aspects: food preparation and feeding. Food preparation is a process. It is easy to overestimate a patient's ability to purchase or obtain food, organize and prepare meals, or maintain a well-balanced diet. This is especially problematic for patients with mild dementia who live alone. They may eat only prepared snack foods because they are easy to open and don't require preparation.

Feeding consists of a complex set of steps and behaviors: (1) finding the dining area; (2) sitting comfortably; (3) recognizing food; (4) recognizing and grasping utensils; (5) successfully picking up food with utensils or fingers and bringing to mouth; (6) chewing and swallowing; and (7) continuing the process until the meal is finished.

The process of eating can break down at any of these steps. When feeding problems exist, careful observation of the entire process often identifies at which step the problem (or problems) is occurring. If necessary, a patient with dementia can be safely spoon-fed. A discussion on feeding a patient with end-stage dementia is found in Chapter 11.

Decode

Cognitive disorder. Because of amnesia, patients may forget that they have just eaten and request another meal. Obesity can result. Apraxia leads to the gradual loss of the ability to use a knife, fork, and spoon. Patients with severe dementia at times will appear to have "forgotten" how to eat. Sometimes they can be coaxed to eat and drink once the process is started. Late in the course of dementia, many patients lose the capacity to chew and swallow. These are sometimes referred to as apraxias of eating and drinking. Agnosias result in the inability to recognize the plate, utensils, or food. Some patients recognize individual objects but are unable to correctly perceive that this collection of objects is a "meal." Misperception can lead patients to eat or drink nonfood items such as soap or paint or to eat spoiled or uncooked food. Taking food from others is seen in patients with *stimulus bound behavior.* Executive dysfunction can lead to rapid eating, even stuffing of the mouth, which can cause choking. *Hyperorality* can lead individuals to place dangerous objects in their mouths.

Psychiatric Disorder. Depression commonly causes a lack of appetite. Severely depressed patients may actively resist being fed. In patients without dementia, major depression sometimes causes overeating, but this rarely occurs in patients with dementia. Suspiciousness and delusions, such as the belief that food is being poisoned, can lead to refusal to eat. Mania can cause both physical overactivity and an inability to attend to eating, resulting in malnutrition and dehydration.

Medical disorder. Dental caries, gum inflammation, malfitting dentures, and a sore throat can cause resistance to eating. Visual impairment may interfere with the eating process. Constipation, cancer, reflux esophagitis, peptic ulcer, hyperthyroidism, renal failure, and liver disease are among the medical causes of diminished eating. Stroke and amyotrophic lateral sclerosis are neurological disorders that impair the eating and swallowing process.

Acute food refusal can be caused by the need to void or defecate. Clues to this are resistance to sitting at the table or constant tugging at clothing.

Patients with Huntington disease and other movement disorders have high caloric needs because of their constant choreiform movements and may lose weight on a standard diet.

Toxicity from many medications can cause apathy and sedation that interfere with eating. The extrapyramidal side effects of neuroleptic drugs can interfere with ability to feed oneself and cause swallowing difficulties. Some medications cause a loss of the ability to taste and smell, impairing appetite as a result.

Environment. Noise, activity, dining area clutter, and television can interfere with meal preparation and eating.

Caregiver. Some caregivers provide inadequate supervision in the preparation or consumption of meals. Others rush patients and do not allow enough time to chew and swallow.

Devise

Optimizing the nutritional intake of patients with dementia often requires a variety of approaches. The ability to eat in as normal a manner as possible should be maximized, but the maintenance of adequate caloric intake is the primary goal. A calm and quiet dining area and an unrushed atmosphere encourage patients to eat on their own.

Patients who have difficulty chewing because of lack of teeth or ill-fitting dentures can be helped by finely chopping their food or having it pureed.

If patients can still use utensils but have some trouble manipulating them, foam handles may facilitate grasping. Utensils that patients can no longer use should be removed. If necessary, food should be cut ahead of time, out of the patient's sight. Patients who cannot use a spoon may be able to drink soup from a cup. Rubberized placemats that contrast with the color of the plate will increase the ability to see the plate and prevent it from slipping. Plate guards help the patient pick up food by providing a "wall" against which food can be pushed.

Patients who are distracted by others or who take food from the plates of others sometimes eat adequately when fed alone. While some may view this as isolation or punishment, we believe it can increase the well-being and health of ill persons by enabling them to feed themselves, by improving nutrition, and by providing a less stressful environment.

Patients who put food in their mouth and forget to swallow can sometimes be cued to do so by gently stroking the sides or front of their neck. If they have a small amount of food in their mouth, fluids can often safely stimulate their swallowing reflex. Commercially available thickeners enable some patients to swallow without choking.

Some patients do not open their mouths when food is presented. Offering a favorite food or a sweet item may start the process. Placing a small amount of food on the lips or inside the lower lip can start the eating process. Some patients who refuse or are unable to open their mouth or allow feeding by someone else will use a straw.

When assisting a dementia patient who must be fed, the care-provider should be seated at eye level with the patient. Cuing helps many feeding-impaired individuals. Cues include putting a utensil in the hand, putting food on the fork or spoon, and moving the utensil toward the mouth. Patients who lose the ability to use utensils can often eat "finger foods" that can be picked up by hand.

Some patients eat very rapidly and risk choking because they do not stop to chew before they swallow. Their food should be offered in small amounts, adding more food only after they swallow. Keeping food and nonedible objects that look like food out of sight may be necessary since some patients will try to eat whatever they see.

Patients should be offered fluids throughout the day. Many elderly individuals lose the ability to monitor thirst. This compounds the difficulties that patients with dementia have in finding appropriate things to drink. Inadequate fluid intake is a common cause of dehydration and constipation.

Family members and professional caregivers should be taught the Heimlich maneuver to assist a choking patient. If recurring constipation is a problem, the caregiver should keep a record of bowel elimination. No bowel movement in 3–5 days signals a problem.

Liquid supplements should be used if adequate weight cannot be maintained with solid or pureed food. Commercially available supplements have the benefits of concentrated calories (most commonly 250 calories in 8 ounces), protein, minerals, and vitamins.

Determine

Weight should be used as the measure of adequate food intake. Charts that list ideal weight by height and body build are widely available and should be used.

BATHING

Define and Describe

Bathing involves numerous steps and can break down at any point. A careful description of when the patient becomes upset and what specific portion of the task is being done when the problem develops is crucial. It is important to determine whether there is a pattern to the occurrence in the time of day, setting, or caregiver involved.

Steps involved in helping patients bathe include: (1) approaching, greeting them socially, and telling them it is time to bathe; (2) gaining cooperation and inviting them to the bathroom; (3) having them disrobe or helping them undress; (4) entering the bathroom, shower room, or tub room; (5) transferring into the tub or shower; (6) washing the body and hair; (7) transferring out of the tub or shower; (8) drying body and hair; (9) putting on clothing; and (10) leaving the bathroom. Problems at any of these steps include resistance, aggression, passivity, and an inability to perform.

Decode

Cognitive disorder. Amnesia may lead the patient to forget when they last bathed or that it is time to bathe. Aphasia may lead to trouble understanding verbal or nonverbal directions at any one of the bathing steps. It might also limit the patient's ability to communicate his/her wishes regarding how and when to bathe or to communicate discomfort during bathing. Apraxia may affect the patient's ability to get to the bathroom (gait apraxia), enter the tub or shower stall, or perform any of the motor tasks involved. Agnosia may limit recognition of the person attempting to assist; of the bathroom; of the tub; or of soap, sponges, shampoo bottles, and other bathing "wares." Any or all of these can cause a patient not to understand what is going on and induce fearfulness, lashing out, or hitting.

Psychiatric disorder. Patients may resist care because of depression. If diurnal mood variation is present, patients may have greater difficulty bathing in the morning. Patients who are delusional may believe that the caregiver is trying to harm them. Visual hallucinations may be frightening and cause distress. Patients commonly misperceive their reflection in the mirror or have other illusions.

Medical disorders. A rash which burns in contact with soap and water may lead to resistance in bathing. Removal of hearing aids and glasses may worsen perception and increase behavioral problems. If possible, remove them only to wash face and hair. Pain and shortness of breath secondary to medical problems may worsen during transfer or movement.

Environment. Cold, noisy, brightly lighted, or institutional-appearing bathrooms may contribute to patient distress.

Caregiver. The patient may have difficulty understanding verbal instructions or be receiving instructions from several caregivers simultaneously. The caregiver may be rushing the patient or be unfamiliar with new bathing routines. A care provider of the opposite sex who is perceived as a stranger is more likely to induce problems.

Devise

Depression, delusions and hallucinations, should be treated as discussed in Chapter 8. Medical conditions should also be treated and unnecessary medication should be stopped. Caregivers may have to be educated as to how to develop and follow a routine tailored to each specific patient. Caregivers who are familiar to the ill person, whether they are professional or family, are usually more successful.

Bathing goes best if the process is planned out ahead of time. Bathing should be provided in as consistent a manner as possible. It should be done at the time of day determined to be best for the patient, not when most convenient for the staff. It is important to be flexible and to allow patients to bathe less frequently or to bathe at different times of day if this is their wish. Being prepared means laying out supplies ahead of time. Before bathing, be casual and social. Smiling and using nonconfrontative body language can diminish the patient's feeling of being threatened or cornered. Nonthreatening statements such as, "I'd like to help you freshen up before your visitors come" may be more successful than arguing with patients who maintain that they have just bathed and do not need the assistance of anyone. If they are adamant that they have just bathed, it might help to ask them whether they enjoyed the experience, all the while accompanying them to the bathroom. It is often impossible to convince someone they have not bathed for several days. Caregivers should not have to leave to gather towels or soap since this could place the ill person in danger, be upsetting, precipitate wandering, or frighten them. We recommend not having clothes visible since they can become a cue for the patient to dress before entering the tub. Allowing sufficient time to bathe provides a calmer and less hectic environment.

For many patients, being in a strange bathroom with a lot of echo and confusing sound is overwhelming. Getting patients undressed and into a robe in their own room can be helpful. Clothing, once taken off, should be put out of sight if possible. Showing a robe and slippers to a patient indicates that the process of undressing is about to begin. The patient should be assisted only as much as is necessary. Unnecessary dressing and undressing should be eliminated.

Ideally, the bathing area should look like a bathroom. Home-like cues such as attractive towels or bath mats can help. A chair should be available to help patients sit down and take off footwear.

The temperature of the shower, tub room, or bathroom should be comfortable and patients should be kept in a robe until immediately before the bathing process begins. If possible and safe, in order to eliminate confusing sounds, the bath water should be drawn and the faucet turned off before the patient enters the room. Patients who are frightened of stepping into the tub can be helped by guiding their hand to touch the water before they step in, and by using bubble bath. A hand-held showerhead on a flexible extension helps avoid getting water in patients' faces. If they can hold the nozzle, they may feel in control of the process.

A colorful floor mat at the entrance of the tub or shower can make stepping into the tub or shower easier. The patient can be invited to "step onto the yellow square" rather than to get into the shower. For patients who are unsteady on their feet or seem afraid of falling, a tub bench or shower bench can provide security. Since these are almost white (the same color as the shower), they are often misperceived by patients. Draping the bench with a colorful towel will give the patient a target and provide warmth and comfort. Handrails can also assist in guiding the patient into the tub or shower.

It is often helpful to offer patients a washcloth and begin the motions of washing so that they can participate in the task. For patients who resist soap or are frightened by it, bathing lotions that can be put in tub water are helpful. Ideally, only one caregiver will talk to the patient and do the bathing. Hair should be washed with nonstinging shampoos like those used with children. Since the process of hair washing is often frightening to patients, shampooing in a setting that looks like a barbershop or beauty shop might be helpful. Plastic hoods that direct water away from the eyes can be purchased.

Before transferring patients out of the tub, be sure to have the patients' attention and to turn off the water. Patients should be assisted out of the tub or shower one step at a time. A nearby robe will allow the patient to be covered quickly. A nearby chair will help the patient feel comfortable while the drying process is completed. Grooming aids (combs, brushes, toothbrushes) that are immediately available can be used to occupy patients until the process is over.

For some patients, a bed bath is less threatening than a tub. With an appropriate room temperature and a calm caregiver, it can also be very soothing. It sometimes works best to keep the patient covered with a bath blanket or flannel sheet and only uncover the limb or body part that is being washed. If this is comfortable for the patient, each body part should be washed and then covered before moving to the next body part.

Occasionally, patients will respond better to instructions to bathe from an unfamiliar caregiver rather than their usual companion. This is most often the case when a child must bathe a parent of the opposite sex. Sometimes a nursing assistant or male aide can be more directive with patients than their own family. A nursing assistant who can come in several times a week to take over this very challenging task can eliminate an emotional and physical struggle for the patient and provide respite for the caregiver.

Determine

Realistic goals must be set regarding bathing. For example, the goal might be for the patient to bathe three times per week without incident. To achieve this goal the caregivers require instructions on how to bathe the patient. Classroom teaching may be adequate, but if this does not succeed, observation may be necessary. At first another caregiver may be the observer. For those residing at home, an in-house occupational therapy evaluation may be used to observe and offer advice with bathing. Alternatively, the interaction could be videotaped and reviewed by an expert dementia-care clinician. Typically, intervention to improve bathing problems is successful within 1–2 weeks. If this is not the case, alternative intervention should be planned and attempted.

INCONTINENCE—PROBLEMS WITH TOILETING

Define and Describe

Incontinence is the discharge of urine or stool (or both) in an inappropriate place—that is, not in a toilet. It is a distressing symptom to the caregiver and often to the patient. It can be a source of discomfort (to the patient), danger (slipping in urine), skin infection, and embarrassment. It also increases the likelihood of institutionalization. A helpful description includes what happens (for example, dribbling of urine, sudden loss of urine), where it happens (for example, on the way to the bathroom), how often it happens (for example, several times daily or infrequently), and when it occurs (for example, only at night). Urinary and fecal incontinence are often due to different factors and should be considered separately. Some patients, almost always males, will urinate in an inappropriate place, such as in a wastebasket. Some caregivers interpret this as a defiant gesture, but, as discussed below, this behavior almost always results from some aspect of the dementing disease.

A good understanding of a patient's ability to proceed with usual toileting is also needed. If possible, the clinician should seek to personally observe (or have a caregiver report) the patient's performance at each of the steps involved in toileting. Are they able to recognize an internal signal of the need to toilet? If not, how do they respond to a regular reminder of a need to toilet? Can they distinguish a bathroom from inappropriate places to void? Can they identify a toilet bowl? Can they move swiftly enough to the toilet? Can they position themselves properly to toilet? Can they lift a lid? Can they manipulate and remove their clothing? Can they sit properly? Can they toilet and wipe? What do they do afterward—that is, can they put their clothes back on, wash their hands, and find their way out of the bathroom?

Decode

Cognitive disorder. Amnesia and visuospatial misperception may cause the patient to be unable to find the bathroom. Aphasia can interfere with the ability to communicate the need to go to the bathroom. Apraxia can cause an inability to lower a zipper, remove clothing, or sit down on the toilet. Visuospatial impairment (agnosia) may cause misperception of the toilet and result in urinating on the floor rather than into the toilet or being unable to sit on the toilet without help. In many dementias, particularly in later stages, the brain (*neural*) control of urination becomes impaired because the brain pathways that control continence are destroyed. Marked apathy may cause some patients to ignore the signals to toilet. Some very agnosic patients do not recognize feces and may play with it or carry it around. In addition, some patients become frightened when seeing their reflection in the bathroom mirror and resist entering the bathroom. Not cleaning the perineal area after toileting due to amnesia, apraxia, or apathy places women at increased risk of infection.

Psychiatric disorder. If demented patients are suspicious or delusional, they may resist help with toileting. Severe depression can lead to or worsen apathy and prevent the patient from using the toilet. Hallucinations can frighten individuals so that they will not go into the bathroom.

Medical disorder. Whenever urinary incontinence begins abruptly, a urinary tract infection (UTI) should be the first consideration. UTI's are especially common in elderly women. Often, incontinence or irritability will be the only signs of an infection. Patients with dementia infrequently complain of the usual signs of a UTI—pain or burning on urination.

Incontinence of stool may be due to diarrhea (such as with gastroenteritis), or, paradoxically, to constipation and stool retention. Colon cancer, especially in the rectum, occasionally presents with incontinence.

Diet and fluid intake can lead to incontinence. For example, urinary incontinence that occurs only at night suggests heavy evening fluid intake or diuretic medications taken late in the day. Sedative medicines can make some patients too drowsy to awaken and void in the bathroom.

Prostate problems in males can cause urinating frequency, dribbling, and retention. A prolapse of the uterus and/or bladder in a woman can cause urinary incontinence.

Conditions that cause weakness or slowness, such as stroke or Parkinson disease, can impair access to the bathroom. Patients who are able to respond to the cue to void but are weak or slow can become incontinent if they become unable to manipulate their clothing rapidly enough to avoid soiling.

Environment. Bathroom areas that are not clearly marked can result in incontinence. Bathrooms in which everything is a single color—for example, a white toilet, white sink, white tub, white floor and walls—make recognition more difficult for patients with visuospatial impairments. Inadequate lighting, especially at night, can exacerbate incontinence. As stated earlier, mirrors can be upsetting to some patients. It is common for patients who are moved from a familiar home environment to a new setting to have difficulty with toileting.

Caregiver. Caregivers should not assume that incontinence is untreatable, is an inevitable part of dementia, or is being done to frustrate them. Caregivers should recognize that incontinence is frustrating and demands time and energy. While caregiver's distress may make addressing the problem of incontinence difficult, it is rarely a cause.

Devise

A urine specimen should be obtained when a patient abruptly becomes incontinent of urine. Putting a collecting device (a "hat" or "nun's cap") in the toilet is one means of obtaining a sample. Though sometimes difficult, gynecological exams should be carried out annually to detect vaginal, uterine, or bladder pathology. Operations such as a bladder suspension surgery can eliminate incontinence in some women and decrease the burden of care. Males suspected of prostate problems should undergo a digital rectal exam and/or be referred to a urologist.

Depression should be treated.

An environmental assessment should examine signage, lighting, ease of identifying the bathroom and toilet, and ease of access to the toilet.

If no specific cause of incontinence is found, the incontinence is likely secondary to the progression of the cognitive disorder or dementing disease. When this is the case, the patient's performance at each step of the toileting sequence should be assessed to see where the problem lies. Efforts should be made to identify the earliest step in the chain that the patient can perform (since performance usually breaks down at earlier steps first). This method of *backward training* will assist in identifying how much assistance and supervision the patient needs. Backward training should be repeated periodically as the dementia progresses.

For many patients, a *schedule* that encourages them or reminds the caregiver to bring them to the bathroom is all that is needed to keep them dry, especially when the dementia is relatively mild. We recommend doing this "by the clock" every 2 hours (for example, 10 A.M., noon, 2 P.M., etc.). The most common error is not keeping to the schedule. Schedules rarely help with nighttime incontinence, however, so diapers and/or plastic/absorbent sheeting is often needed when incontinence occurs after bedtime.

Caregivers should assume that patients need assistance with toileting. Some will need assistance only with remembering but others will need to be guided through the task. When accidents happen, caregivers must recognize that criticism is not helpful. Caregivers need to learn to be sensitive to the cues which indicate that an individual needs to void or defecate and to initiate toileting as soon as possible. This provides enough time to assist the patient and avoid embarrassment. In addition, caregivers should be trained in how to do perineal care. Many men are not aware that it is essential to wipe the woman from front to back to avoid contaminating the urethra and predisposing to urinary tract infections.

For those whose gait is slow or who tend to dribble urine on the way to the bathroom, several solutions can be tried. Laying out newspaper on the floor between the bed and the bathroom at night can accomplish two things. First, the noise of a person walking on the newspaper can alert and awaken caregivers and allow them time to assist the patient; second, the newspaper will absorb urine and avoid soiling the carpet or floor. Putting a piece of plastic artificial grass next to the bed can remind a person to stay in bed and call for help or can slow them down and give the caregiver time to come to their aid. A motion sensor by the side of the bed can alert caregivers that someone is getting out of bed and needs help. Sound amplifiers such as those used to monitor infants can be placed at the bedsides of patients and caregivers for the same purpose.

Modifying clothing can enhance ability to toilet independently. For men, the fly and button closure on a pair of pants can be replaced with Velcro. Sweatpants with an elastic waist can be pulled down easily for voiding and defecating. The use of suspenders can make it easier to get unclothed. Women should avoid complicated undergarments such as panty hose and girdles. Dressing men in overalls may increase the likelihood that they will tug at them as a sign that they need to be taken to the bathroom.

When patients are apractic for toileting, it is useful to have grab bars installed on both sides of the toilet and to slide a bedside commode with the container removed over the toilet so that it simulates a chair. These can make it easier to move patients in front of the toilet, and for patients to reach their hands back to grasp the arms or bars and to sit down in a reflex manner. An extender or commode on top of the toilet lessens the distance needed to sit down but must be securely attached.

Some patients become frightened as they get more impaired because they do not understand what is going on. They may play with feces or wrap it in paper and hide it because they no longer recognize what it is. When this occurs the patient needs to be accompanied to the bathroom and assisted.

Maintaining continence when one is away from the home is a challenge for caregivers. Unisex bathrooms are becoming more common in public places but are still rare. When they are not available and a person of the opposite sex must be helped, family members should ask someone to go into the bathroom to check to see that no one is there and then proceed to take their relative in. Some caregivers carry signs with them saying, OUT OF ORDER or HELPING A FAMILY MEMBER WITH ALZHEIMER DISEASE with plastic suction cups attached to the back for easy attachment to the door of a rest room.

Trips should be planned to provide a stop approximately every 2 hours for toileting if the patient is on a schedule. A simple urinal can be made from a plastic milk jug with an opening cut with a pair of scissors. For patients who have frequent incontinent episodes, it is best to put a flannel-backed tablecloth on the car seat. It will remain in place and protect the upholstery.

It is important to have discussions with caregivers early on about how they feel about doing toileting care with the patient. For example, a son caring for a mother who has dementia may feel uncomfortable providing personal care. In such a case, it is important to help the family to plan ahead so they can find someone who will perform the task. For some families that is the point at which they consider institutional care.

Determine

Depending on the results of the decoding and the patient's toileting assessment, realistic goals for a specific patient should be set. For some patients the goal might be no incontinence. For others, the goal might be no daytime or no stool incontinence. Sometimes the best achievable goals are no urinary tract infections due to incontinence and acceptance by the patient of the use of diapers. It is important to remind caregivers that continence goals usually change over time. If patients meet a goal and maintain it over time but then fail the goal 6 months later, a reassessment should be conducted and the goals reassessed.

DRESSING

Define and Describe

A wide variety of problems can occur with dressing but they fall into three general categories: difficulty with what is put on, impairments in how it is put on, and problems with when or where clothes are changed or refused to be changed. Patients with dementia may lose the ability to select clothing, so inappropriate items are worn or colors are uncoordinated. Clothes may be inappropriate for the weather or the occasion. Many families complain that their relative is not as meticulous as before and wears soiled or wrinkled clothing.

As dementia progresses, clothing is often put on inside-out or backward. Multiple layers of clothing and undergarments may be put on and multiple undergarments put on over a dress or pants. Some patients refuse to change clothing for days or insist that they have just changed. Others will refuse to change into nightclothes to go to bed. Other challenging behaviors include repeatedly disrobing in public. This is not a common behavior but it is distressing to caregivers, both professional and family. Disrobing may be perceived as sexual or deliberately seductive in nature, although this is rare in our experience.

Some patients want to change clothing many times a day. Others awaken at night, get dressed, and attempt to leave the home or nursing home. Wearing clothing inappropriate for the weather—for example, going out in the winter without shoes or a coat—places an individual at serious risk. Grooming and dressing behaviors are long-term habits and often hard to change. For example, women who have always worn dresses or uniforms and men who wear coat and ties or uniforms can have greater problems because they are less flexible.

Decode

Cognitive disorder. Most difficulties with dressing are the result of cognitive impairment. Amnesia prevents patients from remembering what is suitable attire for an occasion. Disorientation to season and weather may result in putting on inappropriate clothing. Inability to comprehend complex multistage verbal instructions to dress can result from aphasia.

Apraxia interferes with the correct putting on of clothing and can result in clothing that is put on backward or upside down. Shirts may be buttoned in an awkward manner or not at all. Complicated clothing such as brassieres, girdles, panty hose, neckties, zippers, and belts can be especially challenging for the person with dementia who is apractic. Dresses which must be pulled on over the head and secured in the back with zippers or hooks and eyes are also difficult.

Visual agnosias disrupt the ability to recognize what particular items of clothing are and interfere with the accurate perception of clothing. Cognitive impairment also interferes with the realization that clothing is soiled, worn, or inside out.

Psychiatric disorder. Depressed persons with dementia may neglect their appearance, dress in the same clothing day after day, or seem unconcerned that they are dressed inappropriately. Patients who develop mania may wear too much clothing or clothing inappropriate to the patient's age or situation. Such was the case with a dementia patient who walked about the nursing home in a bikini with a rose in her teeth.

Delusions also influence attire. A patient who is convinced he/she must go home may constantly wear a hat and coat and carry an umbrella. Patients who are convinced someone will steal their belongings may wear many layers of clothing to keep themselves safe. Those who believe they must go to work will dress accordingly. A patient who is having visual hallucinations may refuse to undress "in front of those strangers" he/she sees in the room. When the ability to dress declines abruptly, an underlying physical cause such as delirium is likely to be present.

Medical disorder. Disrobing is often a reaction to discomfort. This can be present when a rash develops, when clothing no longer fits due to weight gain, or when it is put on in a way that produces discomfort. Abdominal pain related to constipation may lead to attempts to disrobe to relieve pressure on the abdomen. Tugging at or removing clothing can also be a sign that the person needs to void or defecate.

Environment. Many patients cannot make choices from a large array of options, usually because of agnosia or apraxia. Thus, patients who are left in front of a full closet to select clothing will have difficulty. Cues from the environment can be powerful stimuli to dressing. For example, the patient who awakens at night and sees a hat or coat will be cued to dress and leave. Patients who constantly dress and undress often are responding to cues similar in the environment.

Caregivers. Conflicts over dressing can arise from caregivers' unrealistic expectations of the patient's abilities and their insistence on dressing in the manner the patient had dressed before developing dementia. Caregivers who offer too many choices or who lay clothing out and expect the patient to select the clothing and put it on the proper sequence may be frustrated when the ill person is unable to do so. Patient frustration may also result from a lack of assistance from the caregiver. Insistence that the patient dress in the same meticulous and color coordinated manner as before the onset of dementia can result in tension and conflict.

Devise

A plan to address dressing includes an assessment of what the patient is able to do and what is truly important to the patient's welfare. Choices should be limited and clothing laid out for patients who are able to dress themselves. Many families clear out one closet or drawer and put in a single coordinated group of clothing for the patient to retrieve; this increases the opportunity for success. When patients need assistance to dress, clothing should be laid out in the sequence in which it is put on. To improve visibility, a solid bedspread is used to facilitate perception of the items of clothing.

When patients insist on wearing the same clothing repeatedly, identical sets of clothing can be obtained. When the patient is in the shower, a clean set can be placed where the dirty clothes were.

Careful assessment for sources of discomfort should be made if the patient is constantly disrobing. Clothing such as hats and coats should be kept from view to eliminate their functioning as cues to dress and leave. It is often best if clean clothing is not brought into the shower room as patients may be cued to redress as soon as they are undressed, before showering.

If persistent disrobing or tugging is the primary signal or the person needs to use the bathroom often, a toileting schedule should be developed and the patient assisted to the bathroom.

In general, clothing should be simplified to decrease frustration in the dressing process. This can present difficulties for families and patients who resist change. Clip-on ties can be substituted for neckties and knee high stockings for panty hose or stockings. Brassieres that hook in front are preferred. Velcro can replace zippers on men's pants, or snaps and buttons on shirts and dresses.

To prevent layering, make only those items of clothing that are needed available to the patient. Assistance should be provided one step at a time to assure clothing goes on in the correct order. If necessary, closets and drawers should be locked to prevent constant dressing and undressing. In nursing homes and other long-term settings, each piece of clothing should be clearly labeled for easy identification. This includes eyeglasses, hearing aids, and dentures. In some nursing homes, when glasses, hearing aids, and dentures are removed for the night, they are best secured in a designated drawer or a medicine cart which is locked.

When patients refuse to change into nightclothes to get into bed, we suggest that they be allowed to sleep in regular clothes, followed by an attempt to change them in the morning.

Determine

Determining if a dressing plan has been successful usually requires compromise in defining success. It may not be worth the struggle to have a patient dressed in the manner they have dressed in the past. This is often a more upsetting issue for families than it is for the patients. For example, it can be upsetting for the family of a prominent businessman to see him in a sweat suit even if he is quite comfortable. Sometimes the most practical goal is to decrease the frequency of problem dressing behavior such as disrobing rather than totally stopping the behavior.

SLEEP PROBLEMS

Define and Describe

The aging process is often accompanied by a fragmentation of sleep. Cognitively normal elders have more nighttime awakenings, more light sleep, and less deep sleep than younger individuals. The average older person spends more time in bed but sleeps about the same number of hours as when they were younger. Some individuals need naps as they age.

Sleep problems in dementia include too much sleep, too little sleep, and a reversal of the sleep–wake cycle—that is, staying up at night and sleeping during in the day. When a complaint of too little sleep is investigated further, it often turns out that the person sleeps intermittently through the day and night. Therefore when problems with sleep occur, it is important to document when the person goes to sleep, when they awaken, and how many hours they have slept per 24 hours. A chart that records any sleep, day or night, is essential to establish the existence of a sleep problem and its pattern.

The assessment of sleep disorder requires vigilance on the caregiver's part. In a long-term care facility it requires cooperation between all shifts so that every period of sleep, no matter how short, can be accurately recorded. In patients who have a reversed sleep–wake cycle (sleeping during the day and awake at night), it should be determined whether this is a lifelong pattern in someone who worked the night shift or a rotating shift.

Decode

Cognitive disorder. : In Alzheimer disease there can be destruction of the suprachiasmatic nucleus (SCN), a group of cells that controls the normal sleep–wake cycle. Amnesia may not allow a person to remember that they have moved to a new residence and may lead to the feeling that they are being asked to sleep in a new and unfamiliar place. Agnosia may prevent the patient from becoming familiar with and recognizing the bedroom.

Psychiatric disorder. Psychiatric disorders and symptoms causing sleep disorder include depression, mania, anxiety, delusions, and hallucinations. Patients who are suspicious can become fearful and be unable to sleep.

Medical disorder. Patients with dementia who have certain coexisting medical conditions such as congestive heart failure, sleep apnea, or prostatic hypertrophy often have trouble sleeping because of shortness of breath, snoring, or awakening to urinate. Medications such as beta blockers, antidepressants, and antiparkinsonian drugs can cause nightmares that awaken and frighten; because of amnesia or aphasia, patients may be unable to report or remember the dream, however. Leg cramps and leg pain in the evening are also difficult to diagnose. Urinary tract infections are common in patients with dementia, especially females, and can lead to sleep disorder. Medications and other substances which increase the amount of urine or act as stimulants such as diuretics, antidepressants, alcohol, caffeine, and stimulants can interfere with sleep. Chronic use of benzodiazepines can disrupt sleep–wake cycles.

Diseases that cause visual impairment may alter a person's ability to respond to the cues of light and dark. These cues play an important role in regulating the normal sleep–wake cycle.

Environment. Noise, bright lights, and uncomfortable or unfamiliar beds, sheets, pillows, and rooms can contribute to difficulty sleeping. For many people, sleep is a behavior that is promoted by a routine— going to bed at the same time, following the same procedures, having the same person with you, using the same pillow, etc. Alterations in any of these can interfere with the person's falling and staying asleep. Having other patients in the room can cause many of the problems listed in this paragraph. Levels of daytime stimulation and activity may encourage daytime napping and diminish the need for nighttime sleep or alter the usual sleep–wake cycle.

Caregiver. Spouse caregivers who have slept with the patient in the past may want to go to bed later (to have free time for themselves) or not want to sleep with the ill person any longer. Such changes in routine can interfere with the usual sleep process. The professional caregiver may put the person to bed early to lessen work or because of other responsibilities. This can lead to early awakening that is then labeled a problem.

Devise

Sleep disorder should be treated when it is causing difficulties for the patient, the caregiver, or other residents of long term care. As with the other conditions addressed in this chapter, treatable psychiatric or medical conditions should be identified and treated (Chapter 8). Environmental management strategies are recommended even if a psychiatric or medical cause is found. Patients who need to use the bathroom during the night should be assisted safely to the bathroom and returned to bed since individuals who get up to void may become confused and fall. The use of inexpensive motion sensors can alert a caregiver that the ill person is getting up. Putting a mat made of artificial turf at the side where the patient gets out of bed will be uncomfortable for some patients and slow down their exit from the bed so as to give the caregiver time to reach them and assist them.

If the person is getting between 5 and 8 hours of sleep with a combination of daytime naps and nighttime sleep, an attempt should be made to keep them busier and more active throughout the day. Sometimes this can eliminate the sleep disorder. Patients with sleep disorder who are home during the day can benefit from participating in an adult daycare center.

If a diuretic medication is prescribed, it should be given early in the morning. Caffeine should be avoided after early evening, and the medication list reviewed for the presence of agents that can cause restlessness. Restless leg syndrome should be treated in the customary manner (with levo-dopa or benzodiazepines).

A bedtime routine should be established and maintained when this is realistic. It should include getting undressed, washing, brushing teeth, and saying prayers. It often requires the assistance of a caregiver. Some patients sleep better after a warm bath, a glass of milk, or a small amount of food.

For patients who awaken at night and insist that it is time to go somewhere, the caregiver should try distraction—for example, saying "We will leave as soon as we've had breakfast" or "It's Saturday, so we can sleep late." A snack given in a dimly lit room may distract the patient and allow a return to bed. Environments that are stimulating during the day and quiet at night help regulate sleep. Structured activity in the evening may prevent patients from going to bed early for lack of something else to do. If the patient is unable to adjust the heat or air conditioning in their bedroom, the temperature should be regulated appropriately. Some elderly individuals with dementia benefit from an afternoon nap. This should be determined by trial and error. It is best to limit the duration of afternoon naps.

If environmental interventions fail and the sleep disorder is causing distress to the patient or family caregiver, a pharmacologic treatment specifically targeting sleep can be tried. We recommend using sedating medications only when there is a clear potential benefit for the patient or the caregiver and minimal risk to the patient. Unfortunately, no studies are available to guide the clinicians' choice of medication when the only goal is to improve sleep. We do *not* recommend regular use of antihistamines (often available over the counter, such as Benadryl, Nytol, Tylenol PM, and others), since these have significant anticholinergic activity and can worsen memory. Some clinicians recommend the sedating antidepressant drug trazodone starting at 25 mg at bedtime and increasing to 100 mg at bedtime to help with sleep. Others prescribe zolpidem (Ambien) 5 or 10 mg. In the past, the sedating barbiturate derivative chloral hydrate was used; we occasionally prescribe it in doses ranging from 250 mg to 1 gram. We very rarely use benzodiazepines for sleep.

If depression or mania is present, the primary treatment is often pharmacologic. The use of antidepressant medications for depression and the use of neuroleptic medications for hallucinations, delusions, and mania are discussed in Chapters 8 and 10. If a neuroleptic is being prescribed for other symptoms, it can be given at bedtime to help the patient sleep. More sedating antidepressant medicines, such as trazadone, or one of the tricyclics may be used to treat a depression if there is an associated sleep disorder.

Preliminary studies suggest that so-called *bright light therapy* may lead to improved sleep. This therapy consists of exposing individuals to bright lights. (A brightness of 10,000 lumens is recommended.) This is equivalent to a bank of several fluorescent light tubes. Further study is needed before this can be recommended as a first line treatment for nighttime sleep disorder. Chapter 10 discusses its use.

Daytime sleepiness can be very difficult to address. Sometimes daytime activity programs help. Nighttime sedation rarely helps. Very rarely, stimulant medication in the morning helps with severe daytime drowsiness if apathy is present.

Determine

Treatment response is best determined by measuring how many hours and when the person sleeps. If medication is used, careful attention should be given to toxicity. If the desired response is not occurring then the medicine should either be increased or discontinued. If an antidepressant medication is used to treat both depression and sleep disorder, and it is effective, the drug should be continued for at least 6 months and probably for 1 year or longer.

FALLING AND DIFFICULTY WALKING OR TRANSFERRING

Define and Decode

As many as 30% of patients with early stage dementia and as many as 70%–75% of patients who are institutionalized experience a fall during a 1 year period. The majority of these falls have relatively minor consequences—bruising, pain, or abrasions—but major injuries such as hip, wrist, or arm fractures and subdural hematomas are common. Falls are particularly common at night and more likely to occur in the bedroom, bathroom, or stairway. Patients who are at highest risk to fall are those with multiple medical problems, advanced dementia, and significant functional impairments. Also, those who wander and are in good health are at higher risk of falling.

Impairment in gait (walking) develops in most dementias and is often accompanied by poor balance. Patients with gait disorder cannot move their feet to correct a stumble and cannot use their arms to steady themselves or prevent falling. Sometimes, it is hard to distinguish a true fall from an apparent fall because patients can sit down on the floor and be found there by staff.

The term *transferring* refers to moving from one position to another—for example, in and out of a chair, tub, automobile, or bed. Difficulty in transferring becomes more common as the dementia progresses and can result in appearing fearful of or being unable to sit on a toilet seat or in a chair. Difficulty transferring can lead patients to sit on the floor rather than where they meant to sit (missing the seat).

Decode

Cognitive disorder. In general, the likelihood of falling and difficulties in transferring and walking increase as dementia becomes more severe. Cortical dementias are characterized by apraxias and agnosias that impair the ability to know how to walk, to cross thresholds, to go up steps, or to perceive objects in the environment that can cause tripping such as loose rugs, low tables, cords, small animals, or children. Eventually, the cortical dementias impair the ability to know where to look when walking. Subcortical dementias impair reaction time, the planning of motor action, and the response to minor imbalance. Ultimately, all progressive dementias lead to physical inactivity, which in turn places patients further at risk of falls because of muscle weakness and bone demineralization.

Psychiatric disorder. Depression often results in social isolation and a decreased activity level that exacerbates muscle weakness and deconditioning. Patients who are suspicious or manic may try to move quickly or to spend more time on their feet and thereby be at increased risk for falls. Patients who wander about are also more likely to fall. Delirium increases the risk of falling due to worsened cognition and to the ataxia and weakness that accompany it.

Medical disorder. Visual or auditory impairments, gait or balance disorder due to arthritis, neurological disease, muscle weakness, and physical dependence increase the risk for falls. Many medications, especially psychotropic medications, and any medical condition that causes frailty increase the risk of falling. These should be regularly reassessed, especially in patients who have had a fall. Shuffling gait can be due to Parkinson disease or parkinsonian side effects of neuroleptic medications. Orthostatic hypotension, a drop in blood pressure that occurs when moving from lying or sitting or from sitting to standing, can be caused by many medications, by dehydration, and by some medical disorders. Weakness, paralysis, and impaired sensation (peripheral neuropathy) and coordination can lead to falls. Deconditioning, weakness due to lack of use of muscles, can be caused by restraints, being confined, or lack of exercise, and predisposes to falling.

Environment. Furniture, throw rugs, clutter, slippery floors, raised thresholds, staircases, bathtubs, narrow passageways, dim lighting, and loud noises increase the fall risk associated with dementia.

Caregiver. Caregivers may not know the correct way to help a person get up and down from a chair or bed, to transfer into a bathtub, or to supervise dressing or bathing, and thus may increase the risk of fall. Patients who are at significant risk of falling should not be left alone. Caregivers who do not appreciate fall risks are much less likely to act to prevent falls. In a patient with dementia who is falling frequently, caregiver abuse or neglect should be considered.

Devise

The ideal approach to falls in dementia patients is to prevent them. This requires an appreciation of the risk factors for falls discussed above and of the interventions that will address them. Since fall risk increases as dementia progresses, more attention should be paid to fall prevention over time. A Mini-Mental State Exam score in the 0–10 range identifies a very high-risk group. Patients who are experiencing agnosia or apraxia early in the course of dementias are at high risk much earlier. Psychiatric disorders that lead patients to move around rapidly—such as mania, aggression due to delusions or hallucinations, or akathisia—should be treated to prevent falls. Medication regimens should be simplified as much as possible. Visual and hearing impairments should be corrected if possible. To assess for blood pressure, orthostatic hypotension should be measured in two positions, lying and sitting or sitting and standing. The second measurement should be performed after a 2 minute wait in the second position. Measurements should be obtained *before* giving medications *and after* to monitor for change. A medical reassessment should be undertaken whenever falls occur without an identifying etiology.

Environmental modifications should address the items listed earlier in this chapter under the text head Environment. For example, low tables should be moved; throw rugs should be eliminated; exposed cords should be made safe. Gates or stairwells can be dangerous as they may cause falls. Doors to stairwells should be locked. Proper lighting should eliminate glare and minimize shadows. A home occupational therapy assessment can identify potential environmental hazards and suggest practical solutions. It is reimbursed by Medicare if ordered by a physician. Caregivers should be taught how to help the unsteady individual in a manner that both prevents falls and protects the caregiver from harm. A physical therapy evaluation can also provide useful guidance. It can develop exercise or action plans to strengthen muscles and improve balance. Assisted walking devices such as canes and walkers may be helpful but many dementia patients forget to use them or develop apraxias that make them unsafe. Occasionally a reminding device can help. For example, on occasion we have used a device to sound a signal when the person is more than a few feet from the walker. Motion sensors can alert caregivers that a patient is attempting to stand and signal the caregiver to come to the patients to assist them. When patients fall at night, it may be necessary to place their mattress on the floor. Very rarely, a chest or waist restraint has to be used to prevent patients who are too weak to support their weight from arising without supervision. However, patients can fall even when watched very closely or restrained. Furthermore, restraints can cause harm or death and are conceptually repugnant.

Determine

It is impossible to reduce fall rates role to zero without unacceptably sacrificing quality of life. For many patients and families, some degree of falling, even if it may lead to serious injury, is acceptable if the patient is allowed some degree of freedom and independence. Therefore, the goal of the treatment for falls should be to reduce the risk of falling to an acceptable level that does not unduly compromise the patient's quality of life.

A surveillance system that assesses a patient's gait regularly and determines when, where, and how often falls are occurring is a must since it serves as a warning system that falls are likely to become problematic. Any environmental modifications should be given sufficient time to determine if they are effective. On average, 7 to 10 days should be adequate to determine if an intervention is working.

DRIVING

Define and Describe

Even when problems are not obvious, driving by patients with dementia can be dangerous. First, situations may arise in which a patient is unable to react quickly to an emergency or to make the decision needed to avoid an accident. Another challenge is that most dementias are progressive. Even when patients with early dementia are driving safely, a time may come (in most cases will come) when they will no longer be able to drive safely. Unfortunately, it is difficult, at present, to predict when driving will become risky. A formal driving evaluation, on- or off-road, conducted by an occupational therapist or driving school experienced with dementia, is at times useful and might help identify when a patient can no longer drive safely. However, we recommend that driving be discouraged soon after a diagnosis has been made.

Dementia is associated with problems such as getting lost, forgetting where the car is parked, sideswiping cars, leaving the scene of an accident, and running others off the road. Thus, during the assessment it is important to ask direct questions of patients and their caregivers about driving. Include a query about "unexplained" dents and scrapes on the car. Patients often are confident of their driving ability and may forget incidents.

Driving is presented in this book as a functioning problem because it is a capacity that clinicians should address and because the approaches taken to stop it are often behavioral in nature. However, driving prohibitions cause practical problems because they change the lives of patients and their spouses, especially if the spouse does not drive. Stopping the ill person from driving can be a major source of difficulty for the family because many patients feel that their driving is fine and that they should be allowed to drive even when it is clear to others that their driving is dangerous.

One reason the driving is a difficult issue to address is that driving has powerful social meaning. For many individuals driving is equated with being an adult and having the freedom to go where one wants to go. Losing the privilege to drive, therefore, means a loss of freedom and becomes a frequent reminder that the person is ill. Since caregivers must often repeatedly stop ill individuals from driving, they can become the target of angry outbursts from patients who feel confident they can drive safely.

All patients with a progressive dementia eventually have to give up driving. Patients with nonprogressive dementias also may have to.

There are several ways to determine if a patient should stop driving: (1) Ask family and friends about the patient's driving performance. They have often observed dangerous driving behavior caused by the dementia. Asking the patients' children if they would let the patient drive their own children alone is a useful question. If the answer is "No" (referred to as *the grandchild sign*), the patient should probably not be driving. (2) Find out if there have been accidents or if the patient has been lost while driving since the onset of dementia. If these have occurred, the patient probably should not be driving. (3) Estimate cognitive capacity: Patients with moderate or severe dementia (MMSE score less than 18) probably should not be driving. (4) Obtain a formal driving test at a driving school or evaluation program experienced with dementia or traumatic brain injury. Some occupational therapists provide driving evaluations for persons with dementia.

Decode

Cognitive disorder. Driving depends on many cognitive capacities. An impairment in any one can adversely affect driving.

Those relevant to driving include visuospatial function, praxis, mental flexibility, and judgment. The motor impairments and slowed reaction times which accompany most subcortical dementias are another source of driving impairment. These include bradykinesia, rigidity, and tremor. Driving is an "overlearned" or automatic behavior. Much of it can be done without thinking about it. Therefore, mistakes are few early in dementia, even when the capacities that underlie driving have begun to fail.

Psychiatric disorder. We are not aware of specific syndromes that have been consistently associated with impaired driving. Rarely, a manic syndrome with grandiosity may lead patients to overestimate their capabilities and to drive aggressively.

Medical disorder. Medical disorders and medications can affect cognition and may further impair a patient's decision-making and driving capacities. Sedating medications can be especially hazardous. Impairments in vision and hearing can magnify existing cognitive impairments.

Environment. For many Americans, the ability to drive allows them to remain independent, go shopping, and engage in social activities. Alternatives to driving, such as public transportation, mobility services, family members, friends, social agencies, and other caregivers, can be a source of help. The lack of these resources can result in driving after it has become unsafe.

Caregiver. Caregivers usually find the recommendation that the patient not drive very awkward since the caregiver is usually the person who has to remind the patient not to drive. Even when caregivers appreciate the problems and dangers associated with driving, patients often resist or refuse to stop. Sometimes, however, caregivers do not accept the recommendation to stop driving, perhaps because it will adversely affect their lives. This is particularly true when the caregiver does not know how to drive or is too frail to drive. Thus, it is important to assess the understanding of caregivers regarding a driving prohibition and to help them accept the need for the prohibition. This is particularly difficult when the patient's condition appears to be mild and the caregiver has not observed difficulties in driving. The issue can be further complicated if there are different points of view within the family. Protests such as, "She only drives to the beauty shop" or "He's driven around town all his life" are common. Families should be reminded that most accidents occur close to home and that even a minor unexpected event, such as a car pulling out, can unmask deficits and place the driver, passengers, and others at risk.

Devise

The main purpose of a recommendation to stop driving is to prevent the dangers of automobile accidents, getting lost, being victimized, and placing others at risk. The first goal is to persuade the patient to stop driving completely. Some patients accept the recommendation willingly. Often the family needs help persuading patients they should not drive and enforcing the prohibition.

In some states it is permissible for the physician to breach confidentiality and report to the Motor Vehicle Administration that a medical condition exists that makes driving dangerous. In other states, reporting is required while in still others it is not legally sanctioned. When the latter is true, the spouse or other family members should be encouraged to write to the Motor Vehicle Administration and report that a spouse or parent has been advised to stop driving. All jurisdictions have individuals or medical advisory boards that will review the recommendations. On-road tests are sometimes conducted to decide whether the persons should be allowed to continue driving. Many impaired individuals can pass a simple vision test because it does not assess for cognitive impairment.

A decision to involve the motor vehicle authorities is a complex one. It should always be pursued when the clinician has a high concern that continued driving may be dangerous. If the patient has been having accidents, refuses to stop driving, and caregivers are unable to enforce the prohibition, it is appropriate for the clinician to consider legal advice. We are aware of one instance in which a patient was driving in spite of a medical prohibition and had a serious accident and was then told by the insurance company that they were not covered for the accident because they had been driving against medical advice. Of course, it is hard for an insurance company to find out that a patient has been driving against medical advice, but in instances of accidents, such as above, medical records may be available through court actions. Advising patients and their families of this example can encourage them to stop driving.

Making changes in daily life so that patients and spouses can maintain their activities and independence without driving is a critical part of any intervention. The use of public or family resources in this regard is the most common method of accomplishing this. However, for some patients, prohibiting driving means moving to a different residential situation. This has serious emotional and practical implications.

Helping caregivers enforce driving prohibitions is important. Clinicians may suggest that caregivers remove vehicles from the home or incapacitate them. Caregivers may "lose the keys" or keep the cars "in the shop," or always offer to drive when the patient wants to use the car. The gender of the patient and the caregiver is an important issue in our experience. It is typically much harder for males to accept a recommendation to stop driving than for females. We strongly recommend that the spouse repeatedly identify the physician as the source of the prohibition. "Doctor X says you shouldn't drive. At your next appointment you should talk to her and tell her you disagree." While the health professional can have empathy with the situation, they have a responsibility to disagree with a patient who wants to drive and to make every effort to keep them from driving. Sending the patient a written notice or writing on a signed prescription, "Do Not Drive" may help. Caregivers can use this "evidence" to remind patients of the medical prohibition and take the onus of the recommendation off of them.

Determine

After a recommendation not to drive has been made, it is important to document this in the medical record (for medical–legal purposes) and ask at the next appointment if the recommendation has been followed. When driving is deemed safe (or at least if there is no basis on which to recommend that the patient stop driving), the clinician should tell the patient and family that the patient's driving ability is likely to become impaired in the future and needs to be monitored by them and reassessed by the clinician. We recommend a reassessment every 6 months.

SEXUAL PROBLEMS

Define and Describe

Complaints about sexual behavior are uncommon in dementia. While this may relate to the reluctance of care providers to discuss sexual intimacy or to a reluctance on the part of clinicians to inquire about it, no studies have found a high prevalence of problems related to sexual behavior in persons with dementias. The most common complaint related to sexual behavior is a lessening of desire for sexual intimacy in the spouse caregiver without a corresponding decline in the patient. Another common complaint is that the patient forgets that there has been recent sexual intimacy and requests it frequently.

In the long-term care setting, and at times at home in the community, complaints revolve around heightened sexual desire, public masturbation, and inappropriate touching of other residents and staff. Although intimate sexual relationships between long-term care residents are rare, they create significant anxiety and concern in family members and staff when they occur.

Because the exposing or touching of one's own genitals or those of someone else is upsetting to many people, a careful description of the behavior is crucial. This often clarifies the goal of the behavior and suggests an appropriate intervention. For example, a patient who is forgetful and apractic may appropriately find the bathroom but then walk back out without closing his fly. Patients may disrobe because they believe they are in their bedroom or bathroom or because they have a skin rash that makes their clothing uncomfortable. It is important that the characteristics of the behavior be thoroughly explored before someone is "reported" for sexual deviance.

Decode

Cognitive disorder. Amnesia may lead to forgetting when sexual activity was last practiced or what the common sexual practices with the patient's partner were. Aphasia can lead to inability to understand the intimate expressions of a partner or to difficulty expressing sexual desires verbally. Agnosia may lead to lack of recognition of a sexual partner or to misidentification of others as one's partner, leading to unwanted advances. Apraxia can impair the ability to perform movements necessary to sexual interaction. Disturbances of executive function may lead to disinhibition of sexual drives or to attempts to have physical contact with others which is not sexual in intent (for example, hugging, kissing, hold hands, or sitting in someone's lap) but which is interpreted as such.

Psychiatric disorder. Mania may lead to hypersexual behavior while depression can greatly reduce sexual drive. Delusions or hallucinations can lead to suspiciousness or avoidance of one's sexual partner. Delirium may reduce awareness of surroundings and reduce sexual interest.

Medical disorder. Many medications have been associated with reduced sexual desire or functioning. These include beta-blockers, psychotropics (for example, antidepressants, neuroleptics), digitalis, anticancer agents, antihypertensives, sedatives, and antihistamines. Diabetes, hypertension, arthritis, cancer, anemia, and many chronic diseases are associated with a reduced sexual drive or the inability to perform sexually. Pain, constipation, stroke, prostatic hypertrophy, and gynecologic disorders (such as prolapsed uterus, diminished vaginal secretions, vaginocele, and perineal rashes) can adversely affect sexuality in dementia patients.

Environment. Patients who no longer live at home may have fewer cues to remind them of their sexual life. Others may be stimulated sexually by other patients who are disinhibited. Elderly men (and at times women) who are receiving one-on-one care by younger women (men) may misinterpret the situation, become stimulated sexually, and touch or grab the care provider.

Caregivers. The sexual partners of dementia patients may assume that the sexual life of their loved one is unaffected and seek to maintain it when the patient is no longer interested or is unable to perform. Non-family caregivers who behave in an overly familiar manner (for example, calling patients "Sweetie" or kissing patients on the cheek) may provoke unwanted sexual advances in a disinhibited or agnosic patient.

Devise

When complaints about sexual behavior arise there is almost always distress on someone's part. Therefore, a treatment plan is almost always appropriate. When family caregivers report a disparity between their interest in sex and the desires of the patient, a careful history is the first step. Information should be gathered about the nature and frequency of sexual relations prior to the illness and where these have changed. It is important to explore the caregiver's emotional relationship with the ill person. The caregiving role often leads to a change in the roles of patient and caregiver, and this can diminish interest in sexual activity. Some caregivers report a total loss of interest in sexual relations while others report a diminution. Exploring these issues in an open, supportive way is an important aspect of helping the caregiver.

If the genesis of the complaint appears to be that the patient forgets that there had been recent sexual relations and requests repeated relations, the caregiver can be instructed in how to gently remind the patient of this. Caregivers may offer a stalling tactic such as saying, "We'll be alone soon, but first let's go out for a walk." Substituting another pleasurable activity may distract the patient. This is one issue about which caregivers must sometimes lie to the patient if they feel they are no longer able to engage in an intimate sexual relationship. It is important to explore the meaning of other forms of intimacy such as hugging and kissing. For some individuals this can substitute for sexual intimacy, but this is not always the case.

Public masturbation is intrusive to other individuals and is most appropriately handled by redirecting the person to a private place. Most patients respond to this redirection but an occasional patient becomes upset by it. One impediment to redirection is the discomfort that staff and other residents experience in the presence of a public display of sexuality. Often a staff person can identify very early manifestations of public masturbation such as tugging on the crotch of pants or unzipping the fly and move the patient to a private place before masturbation begins. Moving the patient quietly and quickly without criticism can sometimes avoid the development of a catastrophic reaction. More intrusive behaviors such as touching the breasts or crotch of caregivers during care or the touching of other residents in daycare or at institutions constitute a sensitive and important issue. If the person being touched or propositioned is also cognitively impaired he or she may have diminished capacity to resist or stay away from the person. The latter problem should always be addressed. It may mean seating the two individuals in separate areas of the dining room, not allowing a male resident to attend groups with women (or the woman who is the object of the sexual behavior), or moving one person's room to the other end of the hallway or to a different floor.

Sexual touching of nursing staff in institutions (or hospitals) and adult daycare centers is distressing as well. Staff should be aware that behavior they think of as being affectionate may be misinterpreted as a sexual advance by an impaired person or that not all touching has a sexual agenda. However, grabbing and touching can have a sexual purpose or be upsetting to the staff member.

It is rare, in our experience, that a spouse will ask for privacy with an ill person in a nursing home. This should be provided when appropriate.

On several occasions questions have arisen about supporting sexual intimacy between two unrelated patients who are cognitively impaired but appear to be consenting. The fact that people suffer from dementia should not be used to deprive them of the intimacy of relationships with others or of the ability to establish new relationships. When a question arises on this issue we believe an expert should assess the capacity of the two individuals to consent. Such a situation requires the inclusion of family members and legal representatives if patients are found not to be capable of consent to sexual interaction. In general, interactions between assenting demented patients may be acceptable if stopping them would adversely affect their quality of life and if family members are in agreement after a meeting with the clinicians in which the situation has been discussed.

Nonsexual intimacy such as holding hands occurs much more frequently than sexual intimacy. This behavior provides means of displaying affection even when the ability to communicate verbally is diminished. Often this reflects a friendship that has developed between individuals. There is always concern that one individual may be exploiting another. It is important to openly discuss any concerns about this type of behavior with the family and to assess whether exploitation is occurring. Rarely, pharmacologic treatment of sexually inappropriate behavior is necessary. Indications include an inability to stop the repetitive touching of residents or persistent seeking of sexual relationships with other residents. There are no adequate studies of pharmacologic treatment and none is likely to be carried out because of the infrequency of this problem. Case reports and our experience support the occasional use of oral hydroxyprogesterone (Provera) in men, beginning at 5 mg per day and increasing by 5 mg per week up to 20 mg/day. Alternatively, injectable, long-acting hydroxyprogesterone (Depo-Provera) 100 IM every 4 weeks or leuprolide 2.5–7.5 mg IM every 4 weeks may be used. Antipsychotic drugs are sometimes prescribed but their efficacy is unclear. Thioridazine (and other medications) can impair erection in males and is occasionally used for this reason. Pharmacologic treatment of mania can lead to resolution of inappropriate sexual behavior if it is a symptom. Some male patients with dementia and sexual dysfunction have benefited from the use of sudarefil (viagra), although this medication should be used with caution in patients with heart disease.

Determine

Clear goals must be set regarding sexual disturbances. If the problem is a reduced sexual desire on the part of the patient or the spouse caregiver, a reasonable goal might be the establishment of a new pattern of sexual relations. This might include less frequent encounters or encounters that do not include intercourse. Such a new relationship might necessitate careful planning, emotional support on the part of the clinician, and months to establish.

If the problem is excessive or inappropriate sexual behavior on the part of the patient, then the elimination of the behavior may be the primary goal. Behavioral modification techniques, changes in caregiver approach, consistent limits on the behaviors, environmental modification, and pharmacologic treatment may be tried alone or in combination. Responses typically occur within 4–6 weeks. Alternative intervention should be tried if a response does not occur. The rapidity with which treatments are changed and the invasiveness of the treatment depend on how intrusive the behavior is. The more intrusive the behavior, the more aggressive the therapy should be.

Open discussion of the discomfort some individuals experience when confronting sexual issues can relieve the awkwardness they experience in assessing the frequency of inappropriate sexual behavior.

Pharmacologic and Other Biologic Treatments in Dementia

*T*he medications used to treat dementia modify the mechanisms through which brain diseases cause mental symptoms. Most currently available medications act by compensating for the damage produced by a disease. It is likely that, in the future, new medicines will be available that will prevent, reverse, or slow down the damage caused by disease, trauma, or toxin exposure. This chapter discusses the principles of medication use, individual medicines, and other biological treatments—electroconvulsive therapy (ECT), bright light therapy, and brain surgery.

PRINCIPLES OF RATIONAL PHARMACOLOGIC MANAGEMENT OF DEMENTIA-RELATED SYMPTOMS

Medicines should only be prescribed after careful consideration of the purpose for which they are being used, the alternative treatments that are available, and the risks of their use. Clinicians should develop hypotheses about the causes and mechanisms of symptoms and use them to guide their choice of medicine. For example, if the clinician believes depression underlies a behavior problem, an antidepressant should be considered. If delusions are the most likely cause, then an antipsychotic may be indicated. When available, published studies should guide the practitioner's choice of the most effective medication for the symptom being treated.

Before starting a medicine for a dementia-related symptom, the clinician should consider whether there is an underlying medical condition or environmental problem causing the symptoms. A common example is the development of aggression due to a urinary tract infection. Sometimes aggression is the *only* symptom of a urinary tract infection and the problem resolves within a few days of the initiation of antibiotics. Consider the patients who become explosive at a particular time of day and only in a specific circumstance because a caregiver is approaching them inappropriately, because they are hungry, or because they are sleepy. Solving the environmental problem will lead to resolution of the explosiveness.

Delusions or hallucinations that cause neither distress to the patient nor harm to others usually do not require an antipsychotic agent. The underlying principle is that a treatment should be used only if the benefits outweigh the risks. Even if there is some resulting distress, environmental interventions may lead to sufficient reduction of the distress without necessarily taking away the symptom. We cared for one patient who would get very upset whenever a caregiver would come and sit next to her. This led to anger, yelling, and occasional hitting. Careful investigation revealed that the patient believed that her mother was sitting next to her and that the caregiver was sitting on her mother. The solution to the problem was for the caregiver to approach the patient and ask if her mother were sitting next to her. If the patient answered, "Yes', the caregiver would avoid using the chair in which the mother was "sitting." As a result, the patient no longer became distressed, although she remained delusional about her mother's presence.

Specific classes of medicines are appropriate for specific symptoms. Within that class of drugs, medicines differ in their side effect profiles. Therefore, the choice of which drug to use sometimes depends on identifying side effects that can be beneficial to the patient. For example, if a depressed patient is not sleeping well, a sedating antidepressant might be chosen to treat the depression and to improve sleep. However, potential side effects may direct the clinician away from certain drugs. Antidepressants that caused a drop in blood pressure are usually not the first choice to treat patients who are at high risk of falling or are prone to orthostatic hypotension—for example, those with Parkinson disease.

Once the choices of a target symptom and medication have been made, the clinician needs a method to decide if the medication is actually alleviating the symptom and to decide how long to wait before deciding that the treatment is not working.

Once a benefit has been established, it is necessary to decide how long a person should remain on the medicine. Few studies help clinicians decide when to decrease or discontinue a medicine that has helped a patient. A general rule is that a trial off a medication should be attempted 6 months after remission of the problem for which it was started, but the progression of the brain disease that is causing the dementia, the development of other illnesses, and the possibility of adverse effects suggest that clinicians should regularly reconsider whether a medicine that has previously helped should be continued.

INDICATIONS FOR THE USE OF MEDICATIONS IN DEMENTIA PATIENTS

Medicines are indicated for one of three reasons.

1. *To reverse or stabilize the underlying disease.* This includes complete reversal of the disease and its symptoms ("a cure") or the arrest of disease progression without reversal of the damage that has already occurred. These therapies generally require an understanding of the pathophysiology of the disease causing the dementia. Treatments that stop the spread or amplification of the disease—for example, those that block inflammation and excitotoxicity—are included in this category.
2. *To improve cognitive symptomatology.* This requires an understanding of how cognitive symptoms arise and currently involves manipulation of neurotransmitter systems.
3. *To treat behavioral, mood or psychiatric symptoms associated with dementia.* This includes treatments that have been developed without a clear understanding of their pathophysiology.

TREATING THE UNDERLYING DISEASE

The development of these treatments depends on identifying the primary or contributing cause of the dementia syndrome. The ideal treatment would arrest the disease and lead to a full recovery. Examples include replacing vitamin B_{12} when it is deficient, replacing thyroxin in hypothyroidism, and treating a chronic CNS infection with an antibiotic. When significant neuronal damage has occurred, however, treatments often arrest the underlying pathophysiology but do not reverse the dementia. Replacing vitamin B_{12} in pernicious anemia, surgically removing a subdural hematoma, and placing a shunt to reduce intercranial pressure for normal pressure hydrocephalus are common examples of therapies that often lead to partial or full recovery.

Reduction of risk factors is another strategy that can slow the progression of the disease but not necessarily reverse it. The best example of this is stroke, where the presumed pathophysiology involves loss of blood supply to select areas of the brain. Improving blood supply to the brain by stabilizing atrial fibrillation, reducing serum cholesterol, surgically removing sources of emboli by carotid endarterectomy, or lessening the risk of blood clot formation by anticoagulation with warfarin or aspirin slows the progression of vascular dementia. Presumably, these treatments reduce the progression (or development) of multi-infarct dementia.

Several agents are being investigated that may reduce the amplification of neurologic injury and thereby slow the progression of the dementia. Estrogen replacement in postmenopausal women may delay onset and slow the progression of Alzheimer disease. Likewise, naturally occurring antioxidants such as vitamin E, synthetic antioxidants such as lazaroid compounds, anti-inflammatory agents such as nonsteroidal anti-inflammatory drugs-NSAIDS (ibuprofen, indomethacin, and others, and possibly the newer cyclooxygenase-2 inhibitors), and hydrocortisone, and general neuroprotective agents such as calcium channel blockers may prevent development, slow or stop progression, or even partially reverse the damage in Alzheimer disease and other degenerative dementias. The antioxidants presumably act by reducing damage to neighboring neurons caused by the release of oxidative molecules in the process of neurologic injury. The anti-inflammatory agents act to reduce the inflammatory responses to injured brain cells, and some may directly interfere with the pathophysiology of Alzheimer disease. Neuroprotective agents protect cells by stabilizing calcium influx and reducing excitotoxic damage. The efficacy of neuronal growth factors in stabilizing injured neurons is also being investigated.

At present none of these latter approaches has been proven conclusively effective and none is approved by the United States Food and Drug Administration. Nonetheless, women with Alzheimer disease who are postmenopausal should be considered candidates for estrogen replacement therapy because this may reduce their risk of having a heart attack or developing osteoporosis. If estrogen is also a treatment of Alzheimer disease, that would be an extra benefit. Risks of estrogen include the return of menses (called *breakthrough bleeding*) and uterine or breast cancer. Since no prospective studies are completed, the dose of estrogen is that used for hormone replacement therapy.

Vitamin E at doses of 2,000 international units per day (well above doses used in dietary replacement) has been shown in one study to delay nursing home placement and other adverse outcomes but not to improve cognition. Some experts recommend prescribing vitamin E at doses above 1,000 international units per day since the risk of side effects appears to be small, but others do not.

Nonsteroidal anti-inflammatory agents such as ibuprofen and indomethacin have been associated with a lower risk of developing Alzheimer disease (AD) in several studies. However, there is a long-term risk of gastrointestinal bleeding and of renal disease. Also, the proper dosing of these agents for AD is not known. At present, these agents are not recommended for the treatment of Alzheimer disease. Safer forms of these drugs (the cyclooxygenase-2 inhibitors) are being developed and are under study for the treatment of Alzheimer disease.

TREATMENT OF COGNITIVE SYMPTOMATOLOGY

Agents which increase levels of the brain neurotransmitter acetylcholine improve memory and other cognitive symptoms. Several lines of evidence suggest that acetylcholine (ACh) neurotransmission is important to the normal functioning of memory. Inhibitors of acetylcholine, such as atropine, or diseases that reduce acetylcholine levels, such as Alzheimer disease, lead to memory loss.

Approaches taken to increase acetylcholine levels in diseased brains include increasing production by providing the building blocks, chemical precursors; directly stimulating the ACh receptor; and delaying breakdown of the ACh that is naturally produced. It is not possible to give acetylcholine directly because it is very short-lived.

Acetylcholine precursors, such as choline and lecithin, are taken up by brain neurons to make more ACh. They are not effective in the treatment of memory disorder or Alzheimer disease, however. Direct stimulation of cholinergic postsynaptic receptors (through nicotinic and muscarinic agonists) is still under investigation.

The most successful approach has been to reduce the naturally occurring degradation (breakdown) of acetylcholine. Acetylcholine is normally degraded through an enzyme known as acetylcholine esterase (AChE) which floats outside neuronal cells in brain tissue. Inhibition of AChE results in increased acetylcholine levels because of reduced degradation.

Two drugs, tacrine (Cognex) and donepezil (Aricept), have been approved by the Food and Drug Administration (FDA) for the treatment for Alzheimer disease. Three additional agents may win FDA approval in 1999: metrifonate (Promem), rivastigmine (Excelon) and physostigmine (Synapton). Another medication, galantamine (Reminyl), has shown promise in clinical trials for the treatment of AD. The latter four are likely to be similar to the first two in efficacy. Choice of first-line or second-line agents will likely depend on side effect profile, dosing frequency, and effect on the behavioral symptoms of dementia, such as apathy. Patients in the early and middle stages of Alzheimer disease (MMSE>10) who do not suffer from comorbid medical disorders or co-morbid behavioral disorders have a 50% chance of a modest improve-ment in memory and function on either medication. Both approved medications appear to slow the functional decline associated with Alzheimer disease over long time periods (years). Patients at later stages of Alzheimer disease might respond but the use of these medications in advanced disease has not been well studied. Patients with mixed vascular-Alzheimer dementia, or with pure vascular dementia may also benefit, although conclusive research to support this has not been pub-lished. Anecdotal reports suggest that these medications may help cog-nitive symptoms in Lewy body dementia and in dementia after head injury.

At present, donepezil is the preferred first-line agent for three reasons. First, it is better tolerated than tacrine. Second, it is easier to use since it is taken once daily. Third, the dose which is likely to produce results, 5 mg, can be given at the start of the course of treatment. High doses of tacrine (up to 160 mg per day) are often needed to show improvement but the drug has to be started at low doses (40 mg per day) divided into four doses. It may be several months before the response is evident. While no studies have documented that donepezil or tacrine is effective for treat-ment beyond 12 months, there is evidence that admission to nursing home or progression to the next stage functional deficit is delayed.

When patients are placed on donepezil or tacrine, clinical response should be rated by at least one and preferably several of the following: (1) a measure of cognition, such as the Mini-Mental State Exam; (2) a measure of overall functioning, such as a Clinical Global Impression (CGI), or an Activities of Daily Living (ADL) scale; (3) a specific mem-ory examination; and (4) the considered opinion of one or more care-givers who know the patient well. If no improvement is evident after 2 months, the dose can be increased to 10 mg a day of donepezil or slowly titrated over several months to 160 mg a day (40 mg four times a day) of tacrine. If there is no clear benefit 2 months later, a trial period off medication is indicated. For many patients, use of these drugs in-duces a marginal improvement and then an apparent plateau or decline that is sustained for 6–12 months or possibly longer. Figure 10.1 pre-sents a flow-sheet that might be used to guide the use of these medica-tions.

The most common side effect of cholinesterase inhibition is gas-trointestinal upset. Both drugs cause increased acid secretion in the stomach (because they increase acetylcholine levels in the stomach). Rarely, they cause irregularities in the heart rate and exacerbations of asthma. They can also cause weight loss.

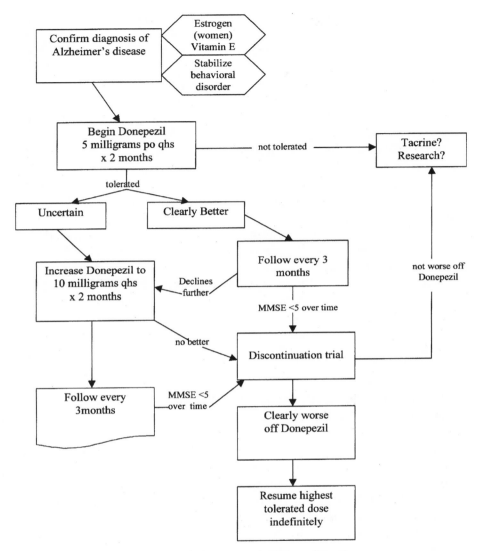

Figure 10.1. Cholinesterase inhibitors flow chart.

Tacrine causes liver inflammation in 20%–30% of patients. This is detected by an elevation in the liver enzyme alanine aminotransferase (ALT). Of patients taking tacrine, 5%–10% develop serious ALT elevations that require the discontinuation of the medicine. Stopping tacrine leads to reversal of the transaminase elevations, and even when high transaminase elevations occur, patients do not appear ill. The current recommendation is that an ALT be drawn every 2 weeks during the initial phases of treatment and, if they are tolerating the medication, they may be monitored less frequently after 6 months. If the liver test ALT becomes more than three times the normal value, tacrine should be decreased by 40 mg per day. If the level is more than five times normal, tacrine should be stopped and a rechallenge considered 4–6 weeks later. There have been no reports of liver inflammation with donepezil.

In recent years there has been a burgeoning interest in "natural" substances as treatments and for prevention of many disorders. To date, *Ginkgo biloba* is the only compound that has undergone some scrutiny and been found effective for dementia-related symptoms. Unfortunately, the one published study included subjects with several diagnoses, had a control group which did not decline cognitively over 1 year (very unusual in people with Alzheimer disease), had an unexpectedly large drop-out rate and found a very small difference between the active compound and the placebo. Furthermore, the compound used was made to standards established in Europe while that available in the United States has no standard preparation. It has few side effects, however, so we neither encourage nor discourage its use. Cases of severe bleeding on Ginkgo biloba have been reported so it should be used in caution in persons taking anti-coagulants (aspirin, warfarin-coumadin, or vitiamin E) or in those with disorders that are associated with a bleeding predisposition.

TREATMENT OF PSYCHIATRIC SYMPTOMS AND BEHAVIOR DISORDERS

Autopsy studies suggest that damage to specific groups of brain cells and neurotransmitter systems is involved in the development of several behavioral or psychiatric disturbances in dementia. The best evidence has correlated decreased neuronal counts in the locus ceruleus, the primary source of brain norepinephrine, with the occurrence of depression in Alzheimer disease. A similar correlation has been found between depression and decreased neuronal counts in the dorsal raphe nuclei which produce serotonin. These areas may also be affected in clinical depression not associated with Alzheimer disease or other neurologic conditions. Antidepressant medicines which act to increase norepinephrine or serotonin levels at those nuclei are theoretically likely to improve depressive symptomatology. Placebo-controlled trials have demonstrated that citalopram and chlomipramine, antidepressants that primarily affect the serotonin system, can reduce the depressive syndrome of Alzheimer disease. Another study found that amitriptyline, an antidepressant that primarily affects the norepinephrine system, is as effective as fluoxetine in treating depression associated with Alzheimer disease. This suggests that medicines which augment either the serotonergic system or the noradrenergic system (or both) are likely to diminish depressive symptomatology. Several studies have shown that depression after stroke responds to nortriptyline, suggesting that depression occurring in vascular dementia is amenable to therapy.

Delusions and hallucinations respond to medications that are thought to work by blocking brain receptors of dopamine and perhaps serotonin. Autopsy data offer preliminary suggestions that patients with Alzheimer disease who have delusions and hallucinations have more extensive cell loss in areas where these receptors occur. Drugs which block dopamine receptors have been shown to lessen psychotic symptoms (hallucinations and delusions) and physical aggression.

Preliminary studies also suggest that cholinesterase inhibitors can improve apathy and aberrant motor behavior in Alzheimer disease. Neuropathological support for this hypothesis is currently lacking.

Despite these suggestive links between brain pathology and specific mood and behavioral symptoms, most of the treatment of noncognitive symptoms is based on clinical observation because of a lack of controlled studies. Therefore, the decision about which medication to use is most often based on treatment success for the same symptom in another condition.

The remainder of this chapter focuses on the different classes of medicine, indications for their use in treating the noncognitive symptoms of dementia, discusses how to use them, and provides an overview of side effects and how to monitor them. Chapters 6, 8, and 9 discuss how to fit medication use into the overall plan of dementia care.

SPECIFIC MEDICATIONS

Antipsychotic agents

Several antipsychotic agents (see Table 10.1 for selected agents) developed for the treatment of schizophrenia and other psychotic disorders are used to treat psychotic and behavioral symptoms in dementia. They share the property of blocking dopamine receptors in the brain. For the most part, they are nonselective dopamine blockers, meaning that they block several subtypes of dopamine receptors. This may explain their side effect profiles since not all types of dopamine receptors are involved in the development of delusions or hallucinations. Several lines of evidence suggest that antipsychotic agents are good treatments for delusions and hallucinations associated with Alzheimer disease, particularly

Table 10.1. Antipsychotic/Neuroleptic Agents

Agents	Sedation	Hypotension	Extrapyramidal side effects	Anticholinergic side effects
Traditional: Higher Potency				
Haloperidol (Haldol)	++	+	+++	++
Fluphenazine (Prolixin)	++	+	+++	++
Thiothixene (Navane)	++	++	+++	++
Traditional: Lower Potency				
Chlorpromazine (Thorazine)	++++	+++	++	++++
Thioridazine (Mellaril)	+++	++	++	+++
Newer "Atypical" Agents				
Risperidone (Risperdal)	++	+	+	++
Olanzapine (Zyprexa)	++	+	+/−	+
Clozapine (Clozaril)	++	++	+/−	++

+/− to ++++ = uncommon to very common.

if the delusions and hallucinations are leading to troublesome behaviors such as irritability and physical aggression. However, it is not always possible to determine whether a patient with dementia, particularly in the later stages, is experiencing a delusion or an hallucination. Therefore, it is appropriate, at times, to consider using an antipsychotic agent for patients in later stages of dementia who are aggressive, "noisy," or intrusive, even if a specific delusion or hallucination cannot be elicited in the mental status examination or by history. The newer, also known as "atypical," agents such as risperidone, olanzapine and clozapine, share activity at a subtype of serotonin receptors and appear to be more selective at subtypes of dopamine receptors. This may explain their different side effect profile, which may make them safer to use in persons with dementia.

The choice of antipsychotic medicine is based primarily on side effect profile since all antipsychotic agents have similar efficacy in treating delusions and hallucinations. Antipsychotic medications differ in potency—that is, their effect per milligram—probably because the agents have different affinities ("stickiness") for brain dopamine receptors. Higher-potency agents bind more tightly to dopamine receptors than lower potency agents resulting in the need for a smaller dosage.

The side effect profile of antipsychotic medicines also depends on their actions at multiple other neurotransmitter receptors, including those that regulate movement, blood pressure, heart rate, and body temperature as well as those which affect nausea and appetite. All antipsychotic medicines (with the possible exception of clozopine) can cause extrapyramidal side effects (EPS): Parkinsonian features (tremor, stiffness, slowness, shuffling gait), dystonias (sudden persistent contractions of muscles), and akathisia (a feeling of restlessness often manifesting as an inability to sit still). This group of side effects makes the use of some of these medicines in patients with Parkinson disease quite difficult. In patients with Parkinson disease "atypical" neuroleptics, especially olanzapine and clozapine, are preferred.

Most antipsychotics increase appetite and impair the ability to regulate body temperature. As a result, temperature extremes are especially dangerous. Most of this class of medications also block acetylcholine receptors in the brain and in the rest of the body, resulting in dry mouth, blurred vision, urinary retention, and constipation. Anticholinergic blockade is of particular concern in patients with dementia since it can worsen memory and other cognitive functions.

The blockade of acetylcholine and histamine receptors causes sedation. This can be beneficial in patients with dementia who have a sleep disturbance, but because of their other side effects, antipsychotics should not be prescribed if sleep difficulty is the only problem. Blockade of norepinephrine receptors can lead to hypotension, particularly orthostatic hypotension (a significant drop in blood pressure with dizziness when arising from lying or sitting). Orthostasis is of particular concern in patients with dementia who are debilitated since it can lead to falls and serious injuries.

Less common side effects include skin rash, inflammation of the liver, and seizures (because these agents lower the seizure threshold). Rarely, patients develop a life threatening complication called *neuroleptic malignant syndrome* (NMS), which is characterized by high fever, stiffness, and delirium.

Long term use of drugs that block dopamine receptors can lead to the development of *tardive dyskinesia* (TD). TD is characterized by involuntary movements, most commonly affecting the face, cheeks, and tongue, but also involving the limbs and trunk. Tardive dyskinesia is irreversible in 50% of individuals and can be quite disfiguring. It is often first noticed when the dose of the antipsychotic agent is lowered or discontinued. Therefore, the continued use of an antipsychotic agent should be based on a careful assessment of its benefit and risks. If TD develops, neuroleptics should be continued only if there is no alternative, if the benefits achieved are substantial, and if the risk of harm that would result from not taking the drug is significant. Such a decision should involve careful discussion with the patient and other decision-makers who represent the patient. Clozapine does not appear to be a cause of tardive dyskinesia.

Table 10.2 also lists the common side effects of the different antipsychotic agents. Higher-potency agents are more likely to cause extrapyramidal side effects and less likely to cause anticholinergic side effects. The reverse is true for lower-potency agents, but they have a higher propensity of inducing hypotension. Newer agents such as risperidone, olanzapine, and clozapine are listed separately—in Table 10.1—because they have slightly different receptor site blockage profiles. Risperidone and clozapine have been studied most recently in patients with dementia and have been shown to have efficacy for psychosis, aggression, and agitation. All newer agents, especially clozapine, are useful in patients who have extrapyramidal symptoms such as those who suffer from Parkinson disease or diffuse Lewy body dementia, as they are less likely to cause parkinsonism. An advantage of clozapine is that it is not known to cause tardive dyskinesia. However, clozapine is associated with a risk of bone marrow suppression; therefore, it is necessary to monitor white blood cells weekly for several months and every other week thereafter.

Many neuroleptics have been shown to improve psychosis, aggression and agitation in patients with dementia. The newer agents, risperidone and olanzapine, are the drugs of choice of many practitioners because they are less likely to cause extrapyramidal symptoms and possibly less likely to cause tardive dyskinesia. Because they cost more than older agents, such as haloperidol, thiothixene and perphenazine but are no more effective, we begin with haloperidol when cost is an issue.

Before starting an antipsychotic, the clinician should assess the patient for symptoms of parkinsonism and check blood pressure lying down and standing. These assessments should be repeated regularly, especially after dose increases. When treating a patient with dementia with an antipsychotic agent (for indications with specific behavior problems see Chapter 8), we typically choose risperidone or olanzapine as a first-line agent.

The starting dose of risperidone is 0.5 mg/day at bedtime or 0.25 mg at bedtime in late-stage disease or if the patient is frail. The starting dose of olanzapine is 2.5 mg. Both medications can be increased by the starting amount weekly. Doses of risperidone over 3 mg/day or olanzapine over 10 mg/day rarely produce greater benefit than lower doses. Thioridazine is a good second line agent and is preferred when the patient is also not sleeping well, given its sedating properties. The starting dose in patients with milder dementia is 25 mg po at bedtime and in more severe dementia 10 mg at bedtime. This may be increased by 25 mg (10 mg in late disease) per day every 4–7 days as tolerated. It can also be prescribed in divided doses so as to focus its activity on particular times of day, such as late afternoon, when the problem behavior is more likely to occur. Although we have used doses as high as 200 mg

Table 10.2. Antidepressants and their Side Effects

Agents	"Serotonergic" side effects	Anticholinergic side effects	Sedation	Blood Pressure	Cardiac Arrhythmias	O.D. Risks
Tricyclics: Tertiary						
Amitriptyline (Elavil)	+	++++	+++	↓↓	Yes	High
Imipramine (Tofranil)	+	+++	+++	↓↓	Yes	High
Tricyclics: Secondary						
Nortriptyline (Pamelor)	+	++	++	↓	Yes	High
Desipramine (Norpramin)	+	++	++	↓	Yes	High
SSRI						
Sertraline (Zoloft)	++++	o	+	o	No	Low
Fluoxetine (Prozac)	++++	o	+/o	o	No	Low
Paroxetine (Paxil)	++++	+/o	+	o	No	Low
Fluvoxamine (Luvox)	++++	o	++	o	No	Low
Other Agents						
Venlafaxine (Effexor)	++	++	+	↑	No	Low
Trazodone (Desyrel)	++	++	+++	o	No	Low
Nefazodone (Serzone)	++	++	+++	o	No	Low
Bupropion (Wellbutrin)	+++	+++	+/o	↑	Yes	Low
Monoamine Oxidase Inhibitors						
Tranylcypromine (Parnate)	++	++	++	↓↓	Yes	High

+/o to ++++: uncommon to very common;
o: not reported to occur;
↓ or ↓↓: reduce or greatly reduce;
↑: increase.

per day in dementia patients, most patients respond to doses in the 50–75 mg range. Thioridazine has significant anticholinergic activity, so monitoring for delirium and worsening of cognition is a must.

The starting dose for haloperidol, an alternative second line medicine in dementia, is 0.5 mg daily in less severe and 0.25 mg daily in severe dementia. We prefer to use this medication when patients are sleeping well, but are very driven or are moving a lot. Increases of 0.5 mg per day are well tolerated with best response at 2–4 mg. Rarely are doses higher than 10 mg/day needed.

Antidepressant Agents

The major indication for the use of antidepressants in patients with dementia is depressive mood disorder. Antidepressants, particularly those that inhibit serotonin reuptake (SSRIs), have also been used in dementia to treat obsessive-compulsive symptomatology and a wide range of behavior disturbances. Anecdotal case series and clinical experience also indicate that some antidepressants, especially bupropion and the SSRI's, can diminish aggressive, disinhibited, intrusive, and hyperoral/stimulus-bound behaviors. Trazodone has been used with some success in treating anticipatory anxiety and in preventing catastrophic reactions (see Glossary). Finally, since trazodone and nefazodone are highly sedating and have relatively few other side effects, they are excellent first choice agents for sleep disturbance in dementia patients.

Side effect profile also guides the choice of antidepressant. Table 10.2 lists select medications and their common side effects for five groups of antidepressant. The first two groups are the *tricyclic antidepressants*, including both tertiary and secondary amines. Next is the selective serotonin reuptake inhibitors, abbreviated (*SSRI*). Next is a heterogeneous group of other agents referred to as "*atypical.*" Last is the monoamine oxidase inhibitors, which require that the patient eat a diet low in tyramine.

The mechanism of action of antidepressants is believed to be the augmentation of norepinephrine and/or serotonin, and in some cases dopamine. However, many agents effect other receptors, including the acetylcholine and alpha- and beta-adrenergic receptors; these account for many of the effects on the cardiovascular system. The *serotonergic* side effects are due to overactivity of serotonin systems and include gastrointestinal side effects (nausea, stomach upset, acid hypersecretion, and diarrhea), tremor, headaches, restlessness and insomnia. As with other medications, antidepressants carry the potential for developing rashes, liver inflammation, and bone marrow suppression; patients are more likely to fall. They may lower seizure threshold and thus increase the risk of seizure.

A *serotonin syndrome* consisting of delirium, agitation, tachycardia, and hyperthermia (high temperature) occurs at high levels of serotinergic overactivity. Anticholinergic side effects are most prevalent with tricyclics and include blurred vision, dry mouth, memory loss, constipation, and urinary retention. Tricyclic antidepressants tend to be sedative while the SSRIs are more likely to be activating.

Tricyclics are more likely than other antidepressants to have adverse effects on the cardiovascular system, particularly after overdose or when levels are toxic. Arrhythmias are due to a slowing of electrical impulses conducted through the heart. Overdose risk is of particular concern with the use of antidepressants since patients who are prescribed them are at high risk for suicide due to their mood disorder. In addition, patients with dementia are at risk for accidental overdose. Because of this cardiotoxicity, tricyclics have a higher mortality after overdose than other classes.

When an antidepressant is indicated, we most often begin with a low dose of an SSRI, sertraline 25 mg, fluoxetine 10 mg, or paroxetine 10 mg per day. If there is no response, the dose of sertraline and paroxetine can be doubled in 7–10 days. Fluoxetine is increased at 2 week intervals. If the patient's mood begins to improve, the dose is not increased until the patient shows a plateau in improvement but has not returned to baseline. Peak doses of these agents in dementia patients are paroxetine 50 mg per day, fluoxetine 60 mg per day, and sertraline 200 mg per day. It is important to keep in mind that it may take 2 months for the maximum effect of an antidepressant to occur. Therefore, antidepressants should be increased to maximum dose and continued for 6–8 weeks before considering the treatment a failure.

Starting doses of second-line agents include venlafaxine 25 mg BID (peak 400 mg/day), bupropion 75 mg/day (peak 350 mg/day), nortriptyline 10 mg at bedtime (increase to a blood level of 100–150 mg/dL), and nefazodone 50 mg BID (peak 600 mg/day).

Trials of several different antidepressants of different classes may be needed before finding an effective agent. We rarely prescribe combinations of antidepressants in patients with dementia other than using trazodone at low doses to help with sleep in patients on an SSRI. If tricyclics are to be used, an EKG should be checked prior to their prescription. If heart block or conduction delay is present or develops, tricyclics should be avoided or discontinued if possible.

Mood Stabilizers

Mood stabilizers are a diverse group of agents that share the ability to stabilize fluctuations in mood. They are effective treatments for mania or hypomania and have efficacy for explosiveness, irritability, violence, euphoria, calling out/screaming, agitation, and aggression. Three of them, divalproex sodium, carbamazepine, and gabapentin, are also excellent anticonvulsants and are most useful in stabilizing mood or irritability in the context of a seizure disorder or in the context of brain injury from trauma or stroke.

Carbamazepine. Originally developed as an anticonvulsant, carbamazepine is an effective antimanic agent that can stabilize mood and reduce the recurrence of depression and mania in bipolar mood disorder. It may be particularly useful in patients who are "rapidly cycling." In dementia, one randomized placebo-controlled trial and anecdotal evidence suggest it is efficacious in patients who are aggressive and agitated. Its benefit in treating explosiveness and irritability is less well established. Its main side effects are gait instability, skin rash, sedation, slurred speech, poor coordination, falls, and tremors. Other toxic symptoms include a drunken-like state and delirium. Carbamazepine can suppress the bone-marrow-causing aplastic anemia and/or granulocytopenia. Careful monitoring of hematologic parameters is important in the early phases of carbamazepine treatment. Carbamazepine can also cause liver toxicity. This necessitates monitoring of liver tests early in treatment.

Before starting carbamazepine a complete blood count and liver tests should be obtained as a baseline. In elderly patients with dementia, carbamazepine is usually started at 100 mg orally once or twice a day. Gait should be closely monitored as the dose is increased by 100 mg/day at 2–7 day intervals until a response occurs, toxicity develops, or blood levels reach the 5–10 ng/dL range (at which therapeutic efficacy is most likely to occur). If there is no response 2–3 weeks after the peak dose is achieved, another agent should be considered.

Divalproex sodium (DVS) *and valproic acid.* Originally developed as an anticonvulsant, DVS is an effective treatment for bipolar disorder and is considered by some to be a first line agent for the treatment of mania. Its efficacy for mania generalizes to manic and hypomanic-like syndromes associated with dementia. One small randomized trial and several case series support its efficacy in treating explosive behaviors in nursing home patients with dementia. Its side effects are similar to those of carbamazepine and include sedation, nausea, gait instability, confusion, poor coordination, falls, and, with high doses, delirium and somnolence. It is a liver irritant for some individuals and also can cause thrombocytopenia (decreased platelets) and other hematologic abnormalities. DVS is less likely than carbamazepine to cause a rash. A blood level of 50–100 ng/dL is considered to be the therapeutic range. DVS is typically started at 125 mg po once a day in late dementia or twice a day in early disease. Liver tests are taken weekly. If there is no benefit, DVS can be increased by 125 mg po daily every 2–7 days with blood level monitoring. If there is no improvement 2–3 weeks after peak dose is reached, a different medicine should be considered.

Gabapentin (Neurontin). The anticonvulsant gabapentin is now being used as a treatment for mood disorder, anxiety disorder, aggression, and explosiveness in dementia. Although several small case series and anecdotal evidence suggest it is a useful second- or third-time agent for aggression, agitation, or explosiveness in dementia, it has not yet been adequately studied. Gabapentin has limited toxicity, usually causing sedation and nausea, and is generally well tolerated even at high doses. It also has very few interactions with other drugs. The starting dose to treat behavioral disturbances in dementia is 200 mg orally twice a day. Doses above 2,000 mg per day rarely add to efficacy.

Lithium carbonate. Lithium carbonate has been the mainstay treatment of mania and hypomania for over 30 years and is used when manic-like symptoms appear in the context of dementia. Lithium may also have efficacy in the treatment of irritability and explosiveness in late-stage dementia. Lithium has antidepressant properties as well, particularly when added to a standard antidepressant that has been partially effective. At times it is used in combination with other agents such as antipsychotics, carbamazepine, or valproic acid. However, combinations with other drugs should be undertaken with extreme caution because of the risk of delirium.

Lithium is said to have a low therapeutic index. This means that the difference between a therapeutic dose and a toxic dose is small. Even at "therapeutic" levels, lithium often causes tremor, gait unsteadiness, sedation, and increased appetite. Lithium carbonate can cause diabetes insipidus, a disorder of the kidneys that results in an inability to concentrate urine. This leads to symptoms of large, frequent urination (*polyuria*) and drinking large amounts of liquid (*polydipsia*). Since lithium can suppress production of thyroid hormones and affect kidney functioning, careful monitoring of serum creatinine and thyroid hormone is important. Creatinine should be measured every 3–6 months in patients taking lithium who are elderly. Before starting lithium serum creatinine and TSH (thyroid-stimulating hormone) should be checked. In patients with dementia, lithium is started at 150 mg po daily. Five to 7 days later a serum lithium level is checked and the dose is increased proportionately to the intended blood level (usually, 0.2–0.4 ng/dL). This means that if the blood level is 0.2 ng/dL and the dose is doubled, the level is likely to reach 0.4 ng/dL after 6 weeks. Patients who cannot be given tablets or capsules of lithium carbonate can be given liquid lithium citrate.

Lithium should be increased cautiously because the therapeutic index is low. One advantage of lithium is the availability of blood levels which provide valuable input about whether individual doses are likely to work. An occasional elderly patient can tolerate and requires a blood level of 0.8 ng/dL but patients with dementia frequently develop signs of toxicity when the blood level is greater than 0.5–0.6 ng/dL.

Beta blockers

Propranolol, atenolol, and other beta-blockers have efficacy in treating explosive behaviors and akathisia but have not been adequately studied in patients with dementia. They can be cautiously prescribed for patients with dementia, particularly those in later disease stages, who exhibit driven behaviors, restlessness, explosiveness, and/or agitation and have not benefitted from other therapies. Beta blockers are not effective treatments for mania or manic-like syndromes seen in dementia. The side effects of beta blockers include slowed heart rate, cardiac arrhythmia, low blood pressure with orthostatic changes, nausea, vomiting, rash, bronchospasm (particularly in patients with chronic lung disease), and delirium. Bone marrow suppression, liver irritation, and a lupus-like reaction have also been reported with beta-blockers but are very rare. Propranolol is started at 10 mg orally once or twice a day and can be increased as high as 160 mg per day in divided doses with close monitoring of the heart rate to avoid bradycardia

Sedatives, Anxiolytics, and Other Agents Used for Sleep

This is a diverse group of medications including chloral hydrate, zolpidem, buspirone, antihistamines (such as diphenhydramine and hydroxyzine) and benzodiazepines (such as lorazepam, oxazepam, diazepam, flurazepam, and clonazepam). These medications have been used for three general types of problems in patients with dementia: (1) sleep disturbance, particularly insomnia and sleep–wake cycle disorders; (2) agitation/aggression; and (3) and anxiety. Although they appear to be most effective in dealing with sleep disorders, controlled studies of dementia-related sleep disorder have not been published. Their ability to treat agitation and anxiety (primarily anxiety as perceived by observers) is not well supported by the literature. Buspirone is reported in several case series to be effective in treating agitation and aggression but double-blind, placebo-controlled trials have not been reported.

Given the extensive risks associated with these agents, including addiction, and their high propensity for the inducing pharmacologic tolerance, drugs in this category are not used as first-choice agents for the treatment of agitation or anxiety. Their main use is in promoting sleep, stabilizing the sleep cycle, and providing sustained sedation for patients who would be unmanageable otherwise.

Side effects of chloral hydrate, zolpidem, and benzodiazepines fall into three general groups: worsening of the symptoms of dementia (such as amnesia, disorientation, and disinhibition), gait disorder and falls, and physical dependency. These three groups of agents share in common pharmacologic activity at the benzodiazepine receptor which promotes the actions of gamma-aminobutyric acid (GABA), a major brain inhibitory neurotransmitter. This has a tranquilizing action on the central nervous system with no appreciable effect on the respiratory or cardiovascular systems at pharmacologically active doses. In contrast, buspirone has a high affinity for one subtype of serotonin receptors and low affinity for a dopamine receptor but no affinity for benzodiazepine receptors. Its mechanism of action is unknown. It differs from the other agents discussed here in having no abuse or dependency potential.

Chloral hydrate. This agent, used in doses from 500 to 2000 mg per day, is highly effective in producing sedation in patients with dementia. It can be used to improve sleep or simply sedate a patient who cannot be otherwise managed. It is a good choice to sedate patients undergoing a study such as an MRI. The main side effects of chloral hydrate are sedation, blurred vision, falls, disorientation, delirium, and worsening cognition.

Antihistamines. There are many antihistamines, several of which are sold over the counter as sinus medicines or sleep aids (SleepAid, Sominex, Benadryl, and others). Diphenhydramine (Benadryl) and hydroxyzine (Vistaril, Atarax) are most commonly used for anxiolytic and sedating properties in the context of dementia and have been used for all three indications above. Side effects include drowsiness, dry mouth, tremors, anticholinergic delirium, and, rarely, convulsions. Oversedation may increase the risk for falls. Diphenhydramine and hydroxyzine are started at 25 mg at bedtime and increased to 100 mg.

Benzodiazepines. For many years this was one of the most widely prescribed classes of drugs because of their anxiolytic and tranquilizing effects. Individual agents are chosen on the basis of the rapidity of their onset of action and their *half-life* (time until the blood level falls 50%). More rapid onset of action is beneficial for patients who have a sleep disorder. In the short term, benzodiazepines can produce beneficial calming and sedation; in many patients with dementia, they can cause disinhibition and a worsening of behavioral disorders. Their use beyond short periods of 4 months has not been adequately studied in any group of patients. This coupled with the high likelihood of tolerance and dependence on these agents, makes their use in dementia risky. Adverse reactions commonly occurring at the beginning of treatment include sedation and unsteadiness. Disorientation, nausea, headaches, sleep disorder, and rash occur less frequently. Lorazepam and clonazepam are the most widely used of these agents in dementia. Their use has been encouraged by their exclusion from nursing home regulations affecting pharmacotherapeutic agents in the United States. Lorazepam (Ativan) 0.25–2 mg per day is given in three or four divided doses when an intermediate half-life agent is needed while clonazepam 0.25–2 mg per day, given once or twice a day, is preferred for its intermediate half-life.

Zolpidem (Ambien). This is a nonbenzodiazepine hypnotic which also has activity at the GABA receptors. It appears to have less dependence liability than benzodiazepines. It is an effective hypnotic at doses of 5–10 mg before bedtime. Side effects include residual sedation the next day, headache, dizziness, and diarrhea.

Buspirone (Buspar). This is an antianxiety agent whose mechanism of action is poorly understood. It has been shown to reduce the symptoms of general anxiety disorder in younger patients and there is some evidence it improves symptoms of agitation and anxiety in patients with dementia. Its main side effects are dizziness, drowsiness, nervousness, and nausea. Diarrhea, numbness, headaches, weakness, and sweatiness have also been reported. Starting dose is 5 mg BID-TID. Total daily doses of 60 mg or higher appear to be safe.

Medications to Treat Movement Disorders Seen in Dementia

The most common movement disorders seen in dementia patients are parkinsonian features such as slowness, tremors, shuffling gait, and rigidity (which may be seen in AD, Lewy body dementia, Parkinson disease, or side effects of an antipsychotic agent). Dyskinesias (excess movements) such as chorea, athetosis, and myoclonus are also observed in the dementias. Parkinsonian features, caused by reductions of striatal dopamine levels or by imbalances of brain acetylcholine/dopamine ratios, respond to agents which augment brain levels of dopamine or which reduce brain levels of acetylcholine. Therefore, levo-dopa (a precursor of dopamine), amantadine (a direct dopamine agonist), and bromocriptine (also a dopamine agonist) can be used for this purpose. Additionally, trihexyphenidyl and benztropine are effective treatments of parkinsonian symptoms based on their anticholinergic activity.

Levo-dopa. This is a precursor of dopamine which acts by increasing brain levels of dopamine and parkinsonian symptoms. If administered alone, levo-dopa is degraded in the stomach and has no activity in the central nervous system. Therefore, it is typically given in pills combining levo-dopa and carbidopa, which blocks the peripheral breakdown of levo-dopa, usually in a 10:1 ratio. Levo-dopa is typically administered at a starting dose of 200 and 400 mg a day (of levo-dopa) in divided doses although doses as high as 250 mg 6 to 8 times a day can be used. A bedtime dose is usually omitted. A sustained-release form of carbidopa/levo-dopa containing 250 mg of levo-dopa is also available because the half-life of levo-dopa is short. Side effects of carbidopa/levo-dopa include choreiform, dystonic, and other involuntary movements; delusions; hallucinations; and nausea. Less frequently patients may develop palpitations, orthostatic hypotension, anorexia, vomiting and dizziness. Gastrointestinal side effects and liver inflammation are much less common. Levo-dopa can exacerbate delusions and hallucinations while reducing the movement disorder especially in patients with dementia. This in turn may necessitate higher doses of an antipsychotic agent which can further worsen the parkinsonism. Thus, patients with parkinsonism and dementia often do best when antipsychotics with less liability for parkinsonian effects such as risperidone or clozapine are used. For patients with Parkinson disease, management can become quite complex because high doses are needed to treat the movement disorder but also induce side effects.

Amantadine. This agent was originally developed as a prophylaxis against influenza (the common flu). It has been found to directly activate postsynaptic dopamine brain receptors. It is an effective treatment for parkinsonian symptoms and produces augmentation of dopamine activity in general. Doses between 50 and 300 mg per day are typically required. Amantadine is cleared by the kidneys. Therefore, the dosage should be adjusted downward in patients with renal insufficiency. Its main long-term risks include worsening of renal insufficiency, delusions, hallucinations, and gastrointestinal upset.

Bromocriptine. This is a dopamine receptor agonist that activates postsynaptic receptors. It is usually used to treat Parkinson disease and other dopamine deficiency states. Typical starting doses are between 0.5 and 2 mg per day, and the most effective doses are in the 5.0–7.5 mg range; 15 mg is the maximum recommended safe dosage. Adverse side effects afflict as many as 70% of patients who receive bromocriptine. Nausea affects up to 50% of patients and headaches and dizziness affect between 15% and 20% of patients. Other side effects include fatigue, light headedness, abdominal cramps, nasal congestion, constipation, diarrhea, and drowsiness. Given its side effect profile, bromocriptine is best used after attempts to help the patient with levo-dopa and amantadine have failed.

Tolcapone. This recently approved agent slows the breakdown of dopamine and thereby increases the amount of dopamine in the synapse. It has been found to augment the use of levo-dopa in the treatment of Parkinson disease. Tolcapone has recently been associated with rare but severe liver damage and should be used with caution and with close attention to its package insert.

Other Agents Useful for Disinhibition, Aggression, and Executive Dysfunction

Miscellaneous. Executive dysfunction is thought to be related to imbalance in the dopamine and serotonin systems in the frontal lobes and subcortical nuclei. Two groups of executive dysfunction have been described. These include the *productive* groups where patients are disinhibited, stimulus-bound, intrusive, wandering, distractible, or engage in repetitive behavior such as hoarding, tapping, and vocalizing. The second group of symptoms are *nonproductive* and include apathy, social withdrawal, and amotivation. Medications which augment dopamine and serotonin neurotransmission may be useful for these symptoms but no adequately designed study is available that establishes efficacy. Amantadine, levo-dopa, bromocriptine, and bupropion all augment dopamine neurotransmission and are agents of first choice for patients with productive executive syndromes. An extensive descriptive literature, mostly on patients with brain trauma suffering from inattention, mild dementia, disinhibition or explosiveness, suggests benefit from these agents. Evidence, mostly from the head injury literature, suggests that stimulants such as methylphenidate (given their dopamine-augmenting properties) are a useful treatment of these executive syndromes. SSRIs (discussed under Antidepressant Agents) also have utility in the treatment of both productive and apathetic frontal lobe states.

Psychostimulants. Methylphenidate and other psychostimulants may also have efficacy as treatments of apathy, social withdrawal, and nonproductive frontal syndromes. These agents are available both in short-half-life and sustained-release forms. They are best started at low doses and increased incrementally when treating patients with dementia. Starting methylphenidate at 5 mg once a day and gradually increasing as high as 40–50 mg per day can lead to benefit in dementia patients. The most common adverse effects are nervousness and insomnia, which can usually be controlled by reducing dosage. Other reactions include hypersensitivity, anorexia, nausea, dizziness, palpitations, headache, dyskinesias, tachycardia, blood pressure changes (both increased and decreased), cardiac arrhythmias, weight loss, and abdominal pain. Delirium has also been reported. There is a risk of dependence (addiction) on these medications and of abuse by others.

OTHER BIOLOGICAL THERAPIES

Brain Surgery

Brain surgery is indicated in dementia patients to treat a condition believed to be the primary cause of dementia. The most common examples are surgery for the removal of a brain tumor, surgery to remove a subdural or other hematoma that is pressing on the brain tissue, or surgery to place a ventriculoatrial shunt to better drain cerebrospinal fluid in patients with normal pressure hydrocephalus. Surgery may also be necessary for reasons unrelated to the dementia and should be approached with caution. Finally, since carotid endarterectomy can reduce the risk of having a stroke in certain patient groups, this may be indicated in the treatment of certain cases of vascular dementia.

Bright Light Therapy.

Patients who suffer from depression, both major and minor, and who have sleep disorders may benefit from treatment with bright lights. The main rationale for the use of bright lights for sleep disorder is that patients with dementia, particularly when institutionalized, do not have sufficient exposure to stimuli which maintain a stable 24 hour circadian rhythm. Rather, they tend to longer circadian rhythms of 28–36 hours or to have erratic, nonentrained sleep–wake cycles. The use of bright lights, in the morning or evening, has been shown in several uncontrolled series to stabilize circadian rhythms and improve both sleep and behavioral disorders in patients with dementia. The effect of bright lights on mood disorder in dementia is not well researched.

However, the provision of bright lights to dementia patients is complicated because effective treatment requires that patients' eyes be open and that they sit close to the lights for a sustained, regular period of time. Typically patients are given bright light therapy sitting 3–4 feet away from a 10,000 lux commercially available *light box*. If the goal is to advance the sleep–wake cycle, that is, to have patients go to bed later and wake up later, the lights are provided in the evening for 30–60 minutes, often between 5 and 6 P.M. If the goal is to delay the cycle—that is, for the patient to go to bed earlier and wake up earlier, then treatments of 30–60 minutes are given in the morning before 10 A.M. at the same time each day. Two weeks may be required for a response, and patients who respond will need to be maintained on bright light therapy for 4–6 weeks to sustain the benefit. No studies have determined whether bright lights should to be continued in the long term to stabilize the sleep disorders of dementia patients.

Electroconvulsive Therapy

Electroconvulsive Therapy (ECT) is the most effective and one of the safest treatments for severe depression. However, there is almost no research on its use as a treatment for depression in patients with dementia. ECT is particularly effective in patients with life-threatening depression, such as being acutely suicidal or having stopped eating. In a recent chart review of 31 patients with dementia and depression who received ECT, we found encouraging results. All patients had a progressive, degenerative dementia, usually vascular dementia or Alzheimer disease. They received an average of nine ECT treatments; one patient received a total of 23. Most individuals had a substantial reduction in depression and 40% recovered fully. While 49% of patients developed delirium at some time during the hospitalization, the delirium had resolved in all individuals by the time of hospital discharge. The average patient gained 1.5 points on the Mini-Mental State Exam. The risks of ECT include adverse reaction to general anesthesia, skin bruises, prolonged seizures, fracture, temporary memory loss, delirium, and, very rarely, death. Given the adverse publicity ECT has received, it should be used in dementia patients only if specialists are involved and much time is allowed to discuss the pros and cons with patients and families.

Terminal Care

Most dementia syndromes are progressive and lead to an end stage of severe disability. In much of this book we emphasize the differences among the dementing illnesses and link those differences to specific treatment approaches. However, the end stage of most dementias is a great equalizer. The problems become similar and the approaches similar. Some differences among individuals remain and different diseases have some distinct abnormalities. This chapter deals with general approaches. It will describe the features of end-stage dementia, discuss the care issues commonly encountered, and describe ways to assist family members in making decisions about end-stage dementia.

THE TERMINAL PHASE OF DEMENTIA

In advanced dementia, all realms of cognition are severely impaired. Memory for recent and remote events is almost absent. Language production and comprehension are markedly compromised and speech ranges from an ability to say a few words or syllables to babbling or muteness. Because of severe apraxias most patients have a very unsteady gait and are unable to walk; cannot feed themselves; and have impaired eating, chewing, and swallowing. Agnosia progresses to the point that patients recognize little of the world around them and few of the people around them. Patients may not look at others even when spoken to. Death is commonly attributable to complicating infections such as pneumonia but malnutrition is a common contributor.

Two studies provide information on predictors of death. The Predictors Study followed a group of outpatients for 5 years and found that patients with psychosis and extrapyramidal symptoms were more likely to die. A study by Volicer and colleagues developed a formula to predict life expectancy of 6 months or less in patients who develop fever. Older age, greater severity of dementia, and palliative care in a hospital within 6 months predicted mortality. They recommend that this formula be used to certify patients for the Medicare Hospice Benefit. The National Hospice Association has also developed guidelines to predict which patients with dementia are likely to die in the next 6 months. It is based on Reisberg's FAST staging and is presented in Table 11.1. Risk factors for death include being nonambulatory, immobile, unable to dress or bathe, having frequent urinary and fecal incontinence, and inability to communicate more than six words. In a 1994 study, Collins and Ogle determined where patients died and the types of service provided prior to death: 42% of patients died at home, 32% died in nursing homes, and 26% died in hospitals. The home patients had little or no home health services 90 days prior to death.

Table 11.1. Guidelines for Determining Mortality in the Next Six Months

I. Functional Assessment Staging

A. The patient should be at or beyond stage 7 of the functional assessment staging scale (Table 1.5)

B. The patient should show all of the following characteristics:
   1. Unable to ambulate without assistance
   2. Unable to dress without assistance
   3. Unable to bathe
   4. Urinary and fecal incontinence
   5. Unable to speak or communicate meaningfully

II. Presence of Medical Complications

A. Presence of comorbid condition of sufficient severity to warrant treatment whether or not treatment was given

B. Comorbid conditions commonly associated with dementia
   1. Aspiration pneumonia
   2. Pyelonephritis or upper urinary tract infection
   3. Septicemia
   4. Decubitus ulcers, multiple, stage 3–4
   5. Fever recurrent after antibiotics

C. Difficulty swallowing food or refusal to eat
   1. Patients who are tube fed must have documented impaired nutritional status

Source: National Hospice Association.

Wishes of Patients and Families in Terminal Phases

Currently, few elderly individuals have advance directives of sufficient detail to guide decision making in the terminal stage of dementia. Additionally, defining for an individual who is severely demented what constitutes good quality of life is problematic. Few individuals can realistically look ahead to evaluate what kind of interventions they would want in a particular situation at the end of life. It is true that it is hard for many to imagine that someone even severely impaired can be healthy and happy. Since few elderly have detailed advance directives, decisions about their care inevitably fall to others—*surrogates*—almost always a family member. Given the difficulties inherent in trying to anticipate every possible situation which will need health care decision, it is preferable early on to have the patient designate a durable power of attorney for health care. Ideally, that person would have an intimate knowledge of the values of the individual and a sense of how they would want their care organized.

In a study of caregivers receiving care at the Johns Hopkins Alzheimer's Disease Research Center, the majority of families were unaware that choices about method of care, diagnostic tests, transfer to the hospital, and feeding tubes, were theirs to make in the terminal phase. Many had little confidence that professionals would allow or enable them to be part of the discussion. Even in the few families who had thought ahead and made decisions about methods of care, those decisions were rarely documented in a letter to an attending physician, for home dwelling patients, or in the medical record of nursing home residents. Most families assumed that "the doctor knows what we want." Yet physicians change in nursing homes, and indeed, those who will implement decisions, the nursing staff, have high turnover in long-term care. In most nursing homes, the discussions about end of life care take place between the social worker and the family, not the direct health care providers.

The Gerontological Society of American surveyed 2,300 professionals and family members and posed the question, "What is appropriate health care for end-stage dementia?" Seventy percent of those surveyed favored the least aggressive level of care. Those family members who had had a discussion about terminal care were more likely to choose the least aggressive level. Older family members were also more likely to choose the least aggressive care. Ninety percent of individuals surveyed felt that hospice care was appropriate for end-stage dementia.

However, a study of 1,184 hospices found that less than 1% of patients in hospice had a primary diagnosis of dementia. Difficulty in predicting survival in dementia was a major barrier to providing hospice care. More for-profit hospices cared for patients with dementia than not-for-profit centers.

The most important way to help a family make decisions about end-of-life care in dementia is to provide information about the options and their likely consequences. The discussion may need to be repeated several times. Question should be encouraged. Ideally, decisions can be made in an unhurried fashion and the emotional implications of the choices can be reviewed.

BENEFITS AND BURDENS OF MEDICAL INTERVENTION IN TERMINAL PHASES

The medical benefits of cardiopulmonary resuscitation (CPR) and permanent gastrotomy feeding are unclear. Less than 2% of nursing home residents who receive CPR care are successfully resuscitated. Even when a cardiac arrest is witnessed and the resuscitation is conducted by skilled personnel, the success rate is no higher. Virtually no one with end-stage dementia who is resuscitated in a hospital survives to leave the hospital.

There is no evidence to show that tube feeding decreases the incidence of infections or aspiration of food and fluid into the lung. In one study that followed 36 nursing home residents for 18 months, no patient's functional status improved after insertion of the percutaneous gastrostomy (PEG). Complications occurred in approximately 35% of the patients. These included hospital admissions and emergency room visits for problems such as tube obstruction (46%), tube migration (17%), leakage (13%), local wound infections (4.3%), bowel obstruction (4.3%), and gastrointestinal bleeding or gastritis (4.3%).

Another common problem in end stage dementia is elevation of temperature. In efforts to determine the utility of diagnostic tests and antibiotic therapy in end-stage febrile demented patients, Volicer and colleagues assessed fever episodes in 75 patients with Alzheimer disease residing in a Veterans Administration nursing home. Seventy-five patients developed fever episodes. All underwent a diagnostic workup including blood cultures, suctioning of sputum samples, and urinary culture.

In 30% of patients the source of the fever was not discovered. The use of antibiotics and diagnostic testing did not affect survival. When they were compared to patients who were treated symptomatically with oxygen, pulmonary toilet, hospice nursing, and antipyretics, no difference in survival was noted.

The transfer of patients with end-stage dementia to an acute hospital for treatment of pneumonia and sepsis poses many challenges. They must be transferred by ambulance and often put under the care of acute hospital staff who are not skilled in caring for patients with severe cognitive impairment. End-stage patients often must be restrained in bed to keep from falling out of bed or pulling out IV's and frequently must be sedated and restrained for diagnostic tests. They are at high risk of developing a hospital-acquired infection because of their debilitated state.

GOOD CARE UNTIL THE END

A focus on meticulous personal care must not be abandoned even in those who are profoundly demented. In addition to the medical interventions agreed to by the patient, family, or surrogate, the priorities of care at the end of life in dementia include careful attention to feeding, skin care, elimination, oral hygiene, and grooming.

Feeding Problems

The issue of feeding is so inherently embedded in the role of caregiving that it commonly presents difficulties to nurses and family caregivers alike. Ethical issues raised by feeding are discussed in Chapter 12. Feeding problems commonly encountered in the patient with end-stage dementia include loss of appetite, not opening the mouth, sleeping through meals, inability to swallow safely, and choking.

Measures that promote feeding and decrease the risk of choking include:

- Lukewarm liquids
- Keeping the head of the bed at a 45 degree incline
- Using relatively thick liquids
- Using a straw with patients who can still suck
- Feeding patients slowly, one sip at a time, with liquid nutrients (once they cannot swallow solids or pureed foods, or using a straw with patients who can still suck)

Stroking the throat or changing from a solid to a liquid can sometimes help clear the oral cavity.

Skin Care

Meticulous attention to skin care is essential, particularly if pressure ulcers (decubitus ulcers or decubiti) are to be prevented. The mainstays of good skin care include:

- Protecting bony prominence
- Regularly inspecting the skin and documenting when redness appears
- Turning and repositioning every 2 hours
- Massaging at-risk areas

Massaging helps improve circulation and provides a way of interacting with the patient. It also provides relaxation and pleasure for the patient. Common places and pressure points that should be inspected routinely for breakdown include the toes, heels, ankles, knees, buttocks, lower back, shoulder blades, breasts, ears, and elbows.

Unfortunately, skin breakdown occasionally occurs even with increased vigilance, attention to nutrition, and the steps listed above. The risk is lowered by avoiding the extremes of moisture and dryness and taking steps to avoid skin tears. Shearing of skin occurs when the skin is pulled in the opposite direction to the weight on the bone—for example, when patients are pulled up in bed while their skin adheres to the sheets. Therefore, it is important to teach caregivers, professionals, and family members to use draw sheets and to avoid pulling patients or turning them if the sheets are moist.

Bowel Care

Caregivers should carefully record voiding and bowel movements. If no bowel movement occurs for 3–4 days, milk of magnesia should be followed by suppositories if necessary. No patient should repeatedly go more than 4 days without a bowel movement and then be given enemas. If suppositories are needed they should be given before breakfast. Constipation can be prevented by providing a diet that includes adequate fiber and at least 2 liters of liquid per day.

Several new incontinence products contain gel inserts that retain large amounts of fluid. These reduce the frequency that diapers and bed sheets need to be changed. Some incontinence products have color-coded strips that change color when moist; this helps one to recognize when a change is necessary and lessens the need to disturb the patient. Frequent checks and changes of diapers at appropriate intervals can minimize the development of rashes and secondary infections.

Oral Health

Oral health is one of the most challenging aspects of nursing care in the terminal phase. Problems include xerostomia or dry mouth, tooth loss, dental caries (cavities), periodontal disease, and oral cancers.

Oral hygiene should include tooth brushing at least once a day after the largest meal. The mouth should be inspected after each meal and cleared of dried mucous and food with a gauze-wrapped tongue blade (to prevent aspiration) that has been moistened with water or a saliva substitute. The tongue should be brushed regularly since it can collect bits of food and infected material. When dry mouth is present, artificial saliva may be used. This can provide comfort and prevent dried contents from being aspirated. Dental caries and tooth abscess cause pain and are a common reason why patients refuse to eat and lose weight. Therefore, teeth that are decayed should be considered for removal.

Mouth care in uncooperative demented patient is especially difficult. Caregivers should never stick fingers between a patient's teeth. They should get help to hold the patient's head and hands. It is important to be persistent in providing mouth care because it is extremely important to the health of the patient. Sometimes pressing between the cheeks and the jaw with a thumb will open the mouth. Use four or five tongue blades wrapped with gauze and adhesive tape if you need to keep the mouth open while providing care. Sedation with a short-acting benzodiazepine such as lorazepam is sometimes needed.

Maintaining Dignity

Measures that maintain patients' dignity benefit them and assure a pleasant environment for family and staff. If patients wear glasses and hearing aids, they should be used if possible. Hair should be groomed neatly in a style that the patient was accustomed to. Good mouth care diminishes foul odors and unattractiveness. Patients should be kept in their own clothes rather than hospital gowns. Women who wear dresses can be dressed by cutting the dress up the back and putting it on the patient. This avoids needing to turn or move the patient while keeping up her appearance.

Patients should be spoken to and called by their name even if they cannot speak and do not look at the examiner. Many individuals respond to touch in a positive fashion even when they do not communicate in any other way.

Roper argues that for each symptom there is a logical treatment that can alleviate it. For thirst, mouth swabs can prevent dryness and ice chips or oral intake can keep the mouth moist. Dry, inelastic skin can be eased with soft mattresses, careful lifting and turning, and the elimination of soaps that will dry the skin further. Elevated temperature can be addressed with alcohol pads, cool baths, a fan, light clothing and bed covers. Apprehension and restlessness can be addressed with frequent stroking and antianxiety medication.

Seizures

Ten percent of late-stage patients develop seizures. These can often be controlled with antiseizure medications but an occasional patient cannot tolerate the doses needed to control seizures. If such patients are not at risk for harm from hitting against bed rails or falling, anticonvulsants may not be necessary. Bed rails can be padded to protect the patient. Oxygen can be given if respiratory distress is present, but this is rare.

Is Dehydration Painful?

Clinicians are frequently asked if the dehydration that commonly accompanies the dying process in end-stage dementia is uncomfortable. This is a reasonable question since thirst is experienced as uncomfortable. Patient comfort is the primary reason used to justify the use of artificial hydration. However, there is little evidence to suggest that dehydration in terminal dementia is uncomfortable or painful.

The issues of feeding and hydration in terminal dementia are fraught with ethical dilemmas. Some are discussed in Chapter 12. The benefits and burdens of any treatment should be discussed thoroughly with whomever is making treatment decisions before therapy is initiated. Some have suggested that dehydration has advantages for terminal patients. Reduced urine output lessens incontinence. Diminished gastrointestinal and pulmonary secretions lessen coughing, choking, vomiting, and a drowning sensation. Electrolyte imbalance, acidosis, uremia, hypercalcemia, and hypervolemia can lead to analgesia and lethargy, and thus less discomfort.

Use of Restraints and Causing Emotional Upheaval

Terminal dementia patients are almost always calm prior to their death, especially if the environment is calm, familiar, and warm. Restraints are almost never needed and should be used only if bed rails are not adequate to prevent falling out of bed. If patients are in pain, anxious, or uncomfortable, opioid analgesics (orally, intramuscularly, or intravenously) should be used to relieve suffering. The short-acting benzodiazepine lorazepam may be used to reduce fear and anxiety. In the rare occurrence of delusions or hallucinations that are upsetting a patient or causing danger, antipsychotics should be used. When medications are causing problems or offering no benefit, they should be stopped.

ASSISTING FAMILIES AT THE END STAGE OF DEMENTIA

All family members who are interested, even those who have not seen the patient for quite some time, should be informed of the patient's conditions and the likely prognosis. Questions should be answered as honestly as possible but ignorance admitted to when the answer is unknown.

Family members should be shown how to carry out comfort measures such as moistening the patient's lips with a cool cloth and using lotion to massage the extremities. They should be encouraged to continue talking to their dying relative and to maintain their connection with the patient as long as possible.

HOSPICE CARE IN TERMINAL DEMENTIA

There are more than 2,000 hospice programs that serve communities around the United States. Cancer was the original focus of hospice care but it has been extended to other end-stage illnesses, including renal disease, AIDS, ALS, heart disease, lung disease, and Alzheimer disease. The National Hospice Organization has published guidelines for determining short term survival in patients with Alzheimer disease (Table 11.1). The focus of hospice care is on palliative care—that is, comfort and quality of life for the patient—and on support. Hospice care can be provided in the patient's home, in a hospice, or in a nursing home.

UPON THE DEATH OF THE PATIENT

The process of caring for someone with dementia has been described as "the funeral that never ends." Other caregivers state that their loved ones were "gone" many years prior to their physical death. The profound changes dementia causes in the patient and the long nature of the illness can result in an awkward experience at the end.

A variety of reactions are observed in family members. Two scenarios are common. In the first, the caregiver is intellectually prepared for the death of the patient but experiences intense feelings of sadness at the actual event. Persons in this situation often express surprise and occasional embarrassment at their "lack of control" over their feelings. It is useful to inform them that intellectual and emotional reactions are different and both are necessary parts of the grieving process.

In the second scenario, the funeral process becomes awkward when the caregiver feels relief that the death has finally occurred. Often persons who have not been directly involved in caregiving will attend funeral or memorial services. They may feel shocked and intensely saddened and be puzzled or even critical of the primary caregiver who does not express consonant feelings. Even within a family, the reaction to the death may be quite different for different members. The explanation that all persons do not have to be at the same place in grieving can be reassuring to such families.

As in other chronic illnesses, it is sometimes difficult to recall life with patients when they were well. Our practice is to meet with surviving family members several months after the death. This meeting is often initially upsetting as it is the first visit to the office without the patient. The meeting provides an opportunity to review the life before the illness and to provide praise for a long ordeal of caregiving. Many families have reported that such meetings release them from the mourning process to continue their lives.

THE ISSUE OF AUTOPSY

In our experience, the issue of autopsy confirmation of the diagnosis of the cause of dementia arises commonly. As reviewed earlier, when the diagnostic procedures we recommend are followed, the diagnosis of Alzheimer disease is confirmed at autopsy over 90% of the time. Thus, the autopsy is not necessary in most cases of Alzheimer. In addition, less typical dementias, such as Lewy body dementia or vascular dementia, are hard to diagnose while the patient is living. Moreover, autopsy confirmation reassures some that nothing was missed that could have been treated. In families where several persons have had dementia, establishing the diagnosis provides information that defines risk, and in the future, possibilities for prevention in surviving family members. When the autopsy is conducted as part of a research study, an added benefit is possible. The information gained from the autopsy adds to the body of knowledge abut dementing illnesses and can thus help future generations. For many, it is a source of pride that something positive was contributed from an unfortunate illness.

Ethical and Legal Issues

C hronic illnesses like dementia raise many ethical, moral, and legal issues. Discussions of ethical issues are often frustrating be- cause they do not end with an expert telling clinicians the "right" thing to do. Nevertheless, an open discussion of ethical con- cerns is important because it alerts practitioners to an important aspect of what they do. Discussion sometimes leads to consensus on the appro- priate action. At other times, it clarifies the available options. This chapter first discusses six ethical issues that arise in dementia care and then uses these examples to develop several principles that guide our practice. This is followed by a discussion of the most common legal is- sues which arise in the care of dementia patients.

ETHICAL ISSUES

The Person With Memory Problems who Doesn't Want to Be Evaluated

It is common for individuals with memory impairment to be unaware that they have a problem. When memory problems are brought to their attention some are happy to seek medical attention but others refuse an evaluation. What can a family member or professional do when evalua- tion is refused? Several issues are clear. It is impossible to force indi- viduals to seek medical care if they do not want it unless the situation is acutely life threatening. As a culture, we have established, and the courts have confirmed, the right of a "competent" individual to refuse treatment. The difficult issue that arises in individuals with memory loss is whether they actually have the capacity to make an informed choice to refuse evaluation and treatment.

It is appropriate and ethical for family members, friends, physicians, and others to encourage and even urge a person with memory problems to have a complete assessment. At times individuals will agree to be evaluated if a family member or close friend accompanies them to the doctor. For the vast majority of people, frequent encouragement, even nagging, will eventually lead to their seeing a physician. However, if a person continues to refuse a medical assessment, there is little that can be done to force an evaluation unless a clearly dangerous situation presents itself. In some communities a geriatric evaluation service can force an evaluation, but usually only when a clear danger is present.

When a person who is reluctant or unable to acknowledge a memory problem has a doctor's appointment, the family should consider calling ahead to alert the physician that this is a problem. This will assure that the proper medical assessment is done. This can also alert the physician that there are important social or practical questions, such as living alone and driving, that need to be addressed.

Unless there is clear evidence of danger, a person cannot be forced to undergo an evaluation for memory disorder. Persistent encouragement can often lead the reluctant individual to undergo an evaluation.

The Person Who Lives Alone

Most dementing illnesses ultimately rob people of their independence. When questions arise about their ability to live alone, a professional evaluation of the many abilities needed to be independent should be sought. Among the questions to be reviewed are: Can they find their way around the neighborhood or do they get lost, even occasionally? Are they able to prepare proper meals? Can they recognize an emergency situation and do they know how to get help (dial the telephone, dial 911)? Is there someone available to "keep an eye" on the person?

Competent adults have the right to choose where they want to live. Most of us would interfere with this right only in extreme circumstances. In a majority of instances the person with dementia can eventually be convinced that the move to a safer environment is necessary. However, when there is a significant likelihood that harm would come to the person or to someone else as a result of wandering, malnutrition, fire, or failure to take medication, we should intervene. If the person cannot be convinced and clear danger is present, then a legal solution should be sought.

It is often possible to find intermediate solutions to a dilemma such as this. For example, even when people are unable to live alone, their impairments may not necessitate placement in a nursing home. In-between options include hiring a home companion, having the person attend a daycare center while family members are at work, or moving to a small group home. These examples illustrate that many ethical dilemmas can be solved by finding a middle ground between two extremes. In this situation individuals may not fully have the ability to determine their living situation, but they can be helped if they are provided with a set of options and then are encouraged to choose.

Attempts should be made to maximize choice, even in an impaired individual. Offering a range of options can sometimes preserve a person's right to choose, but from a limited menu of choices.

Should Anyone With Dementia Be Allowed to Drive?

Driving presents difficult clinical and ethical dilemmas. For many individuals and their spouses, driving is necessary to remain active and independent—important goals in the treatment of dementia.

However, driving is a complex skill that depends on many physical and cognitive skills. It is unclear exactly when in the course of dementia the ability to drive safely is lost, but all progressive dementing diseases ultimately impair the skills needed to drive.

Some clinicians have concluded that any person with a diagnosis of dementia should stop driving because we cannot know when driving ability is lost and because impaired driving places others at risk. Others argue that there must be evidence of danger, such as poor performance on neuropsychological tests that measure reaction time, judgment, or perception skills; a history of automobile accidents; or a failed driving test, before a person should be forced to stop driving. Those holding this latter opinion note that driving can often be the only means of getting food from the grocery store, visiting others, and keeping active. Preventing some individuals from driving may also adversely affect a spouse who is unable to drive.

There is universal agreement, though, that a person's privilege to drive should be revoked once there is clear evidence of impairment in the skills required for driving. It is only in the group of patients who have yet to show impairments over which ethical dilemmas arise and significant disagreement exist.

Because impaired driving places others at risk of harm and because driving is a privilege, not a right, the standards for depriving a person of the privilege to drive are less strict than those for the two previous examples—refusing an evaluation and wanting to live alone. We recommend that all individuals who have received a diagnosis of dementia stop driving and be carefully evaluated prior to resuming driving. We base this on recent evidence that even patients with mild dementia have impaired driving ability and on the inability to know when the ability first becomes impaired.

The recommendation to stop driving is easy to make if the person with dementia has someone else available who can drive. Even when the ability to drive seems intact, many patients stop driving on their own or at their family's or physician's recommendation. Difficulties arise when individuals persist in wanting to drive or if their families feel their driving is a necessity. ("It's the only way we can get groceries.") When these issues arise we refer the patient to a driving school and sometimes also for neuropsychological testing. If the driving school or testing results suggest there is danger then a strong recommendation to stop driving is made. If legally permissible, the appropriate authorities should be notified. If the driving test and neuropsychological tests reveal no evidence of impairment that would interfere with driving, we inform the patient and family that we still believe some danger exists, that driving problems are likely to develop in the future, and that the person should no longer drive.

The law regarding notification of the motor vehicle bureau that a person's driving ability is impaired varies greatly across the United States. In some states, physicians are required to report all persons with a diagnosis of dementia or Alzheimer disease to the motor vehicle authority. In other states, notification is not permissible because of confidentiality statutes. We believe this question should be settled legislatively since this is one way for "society" to express a collective opinion on a difficult issue over which clinicians disagree.

When danger to others exists we are justified in depriving persons of something that they want. However, since there is no consensus on when the driving privilege should be revoked and since driving is a legally granted privilege, the authorities who legislate and regulate this privilege should address the issue.

Should Medications and Restraints Be Used to Control Behavior and Protect Patients From Harm?

One of the most distressing aspects of a visit to a nursing home is the sight of individuals secured in chairs or appearing "drugged." As is discussed in Chapters 8 and 9, patients with dementia commonly suffer from functional impairments or behaviors that are distressing to them and place the patient or others at risk of harm. A duty to protect the ill person from harm and distress is well established, but clinical practice also mandates that patients be treated in the least restrictive manner. The conflicting goals of protection from harm (and thereby limitation of freedom) vs. maximization of independence underlie several of the issues discussed in this chapter. The ideal solution usually involves finding a midpoint that allows as much freedom as seems safe *and* provides the lowest amount of restriction that will minimize danger and distress.

If a behavior in question presents no danger to the patient or others and no significant distress to the patient, it should probably be allowed to continue. (See Chapter 8 for examples.) If a psychiatric disorder (in addition to dementia) is the cause of the behavior problem and the patient is likely to benefit directly from treatment, this therapy should be given strong consideration. When neither danger nor benefit is clear, the potential benefit to the ill person must be weighed against the potential for harm. In general, this means trying the least restrictive nonpharmacologic, nonrestraint approaches first (Chapters 8 and 9) and then trying medication for specific indications. Physical restraints should be considered only for *specific indications* that are identified in the medical record when danger to self or others is present or significant emotional distress is likely in the ill person. In general, invasive therapies such as physical restraint should be continued only as long as the behavior or physical problem remains a danger and the treatment is documented to be helpful or protective of safety.

The least restrictive, safest, and most effective treatment should be chose for each problem. Balancing these goals can be challenging. Not labeling an issue a "problem" is appropriate if the patient or others do not experience harm or distress. Treatment is appropriate when distress or harm is possible or likely.

Is it Ever Proper to Lie to a Person With Dementia?

A very distressing behavior associated with dementia is the constant repetition of a question or incorrect statement. Some patients repeatedly ask to go home, ask where their parents are, or claim that a specific individual is harming them. Among the options open to managing this are *distraction* (getting the person to think or talk about something else), *dealing with the underlying feelings* rather than the statement itself ("You sound lonely today"; "It sounds like you miss your mother"; "Are you feeling lost?"), and *ignoring* the statement.

None of these approaches directly addresses the patient's concern. Rather they redefine it, assume that there is some other concern that is actually being expressed, or ignore it. Directly addressing the issue (for example, "Your mother is dead") is often harmful and rarely benefits the ill person.

Why are we comfortable using distraction or addressing the problem by lying? Undoubtedly, part of the reason is because these approaches work. More importantly, though, these strategies enable us to have a meaningful interaction with demented individuals *and* diminish their upset. We prefer these approaches to blunt truth telling (such as, "Your mother's dead" or "You're going to live here the rest of your life") because they are less upsetting to ill individuals, they allow us to communicate with them in a positive fashion, and they benefit the patient by encouraging them to express their emotions.

Furthermore, blunt "truth telling" does not benefit many people with dementia because they are often unable to remember or appreciate the "truth." Since helping rather than hurting patients is our primary goal, it follows that distraction, discussing facing one's feeling, and ignoring can simultaneously be beneficial to the patient and avoid harming them.

Distraction and focusing on feelings are not lies but they are not telling the full truth either. Unfortunately, there are times when these approaches do not work. When they fail, the ill person often becomes more upset, restless, angry, or even physically combative. Many practitioners report that they will say, "Your mother will be here soon, don't worry." when she has been deceased for a number of years, or, "You're just staying here for a little while until your health gets better" when the person has permanently moved to a child's home or a nursing home. We believe this is lying and raises what is an awkward question: Is this lying justifiable? Is lying ever justifiable? We believe the answer is yes and that this is one of the very few circumstances when it is.

Upset and distress are unavoidable aspects of living. As human beings we have many means of adapting to loss and disappointment. Unfortunately, some persons with dementia are robbed of these adaptive mechanisms. They cannot remember new information, so the grieving process that human beings rely on to adapt to loss cannot evolve as it usually does. Some individuals with dementia cannot express themselves verbally and so cannot share with others their distress and concerns, another important mechanism that can help one adapt. Adding to these problems is that many patients have a diminished capacity to learn from experience.

Dementing illnesses predispose people to emotional outbursts. Some individuals with dementia remain distressed and agitated despite reassurance, distraction, and emotional support. In this situation the *inappropriate* response is the one that further distresses the patient. The *appropriate* response is the one that relieves distress. To our great discomfort, this sometimes involves lying.

We share the value that lying is something wrong. We believe lying can only be justified as a last resort and only when it is the sole means of relieving the distress of a person with dementia. One justification for lying in this circumstance is that, for the patient, the truth cannot be true. A statement that is true for us ("You live here now." "It sounds like you're frightened." "How do you think we should fix the place up?" "Your mother passed away several years ago") may *not* be true for patients because the illness prevents them from knowing it. For them, their mother is still living and this is not where they live. For them, "reality" is different than what is "true" for us. Said in another way, the lie or partial truth that we tell is an untruth *for us*, not for the patient. Since the purpose of our intervention is to relieve the patient's distress, not to convince them of *our* reality, an untruth is often more beneficial than the truth. Ideally all other approaches, including telling the truth once or twice and assessing whether it benefits or harms the person, should be tried first.

Acting to reduce distress and to preserve a patient's dignity is an important principle of dementia care. In most circumstances lying is unacceptable, but if it is the only way to relieve distress in a person who cannot benefit from the truth, then it is justifiable.

Who Should Make Health Decisions for a Person Who Is Severely Incapacitated?

In the United States, most people believe that an individual's wishes expressed prior to becoming incapacitated should be followed, if possible. Even with the availability of legal documents such as the durable power of attorney for health (discussed later in this chapter), it is difficult for people to predict and discuss ahead of time all the major decision points that reflect their views. Ideally, each of us will have discussed our broad desires with someone we trust and legally empowered them to express these wishes through an advanced directive. Often, however, neither of these has taken place. Who should make decisions for the incapacitated person?

Precedent and law empower the family to make substituted judgments in some states. In others, the trend is for legal representatives to be appointed. Which is most desirable? We believe the family should make substituted judgment unless there is reason to suspect that they are not acting on behalf of and in the best interest of the ill person. Our reliance on the family reflects our clinical experience that most families have their loved one's best interests at heart and have struggled to dignify and support the ill person. Most family members undoubtedly consider their own physical, financial and emotional needs when making substitute judgments. However, it is rare that family members consider their own needs to the detriment of the patient's. When this does occur, a legal solution, such as a court-appointed guardianship, should be sought.

Occasionally, disagreements arise among family members or between the family and health care provider. These can usually be resolved by helping family members and the treatment team work together to reach consensus. When disagreements exist, the first step is to review the medical "facts" of the situation. For example, determine what is known about the specific problem under discussion, what options are available, and what are the likely outcomes of each approach. It may take several meetings to cover all the issues that need to be reviewed since most people are unaccustomed to discussing complex medical issues and because these discussions often occur in upsetting circumstances.

In the rare instance that family members cannot reach agreement, it is appropriate to seek help from others. If the clergy have not been consulted by the family this should be suggested. Social workers and medical consultants (both nurses and physicians) can be helpful. All hospitals and some nursing homes have ethics consultants who may be of help. Rarely, the family will need to see a new physician or nursing home because the current practitioner or institution cannot meet their needs. In extremely rare circumstances, legal adjudication must be sought.

Incompetent individuals should be *protected*. When they no longer have the capacity to decide for themselves, someone should make decisions for them. Ideally this should be someone who knows their lifelong values and who will make decisions in their best interests. Family members are in the best position to "stand in" for the ill person because they can best represent the ill person's long-held beliefs and consider the ill person's best interests. Legal adjudication is necessary when disagreements cannot be resolved by time and discussion or when the ill person's best interests are not being considered by those making decisions.

Refusal to Eat

Patients with dementia typically lose a few pounds per year as the disease progresses. In a minority of individuals weight loss becomes a significant health concern. For a small percentage weight loss becomes life threatening. There are many reasons a person with dementia might not eat (see Chapter 9).

A small percentage of individuals with dementia actively resist food. They push away the spoon or food when people attempt to feed them. If food refusal or weight loss develops, it is necessary to determine whether an identifiable cause of the eating difficulty is present and whether the problem can be treated (see Chapter 9).

Dilemmas arise when no treatable cause for poor food intake is identified or when the inability to swallow appears to be lost permanently due to the disease. If weight loss continues, severe debilitation and death become likely. What options are available? Attempts to feed by mouth should go on as long as they are safe. This preserves eating as a "natural" function. It also provides a way of giving individual care, attention, and love to an impaired person.

Most individuals with dementia who have life-threatening eating problems are severely demented. As a result, decisions about artificial feeding must be made by others. If the person's previously stated wishes can be reasonably accommodated, they should be weighed very heavily in making a decision. How strongly they should influence the person who has authority to make the final decision is a difficult question since the details of specific situations are almost never known ahead of time. Some would argue that a prior expressed wish must always be followed. We believe the circumstances of each decision require careful thought and that no absolute rule can be stated.

So-called *artificial feeding* is defined as feeding by blood vessel, usually by vein (intravenously), rarely by artery, or by a tube that is inserted either through the nose (*nasogastric tube*) or through the abdominal wall directly into the stomach (*gastrostomy tube*). A discussion of these options should be started as soon as it becomes evident that a person is losing weight more rapidly than expected and no treatable cause is found. Ideally, this discussion would begin months before any decision must be made. This allows the family or decisionmaker time to decide what actions they would like to take to address the problem and avoids the need to make a sudden decision. Most medical ethicists and courts agree that the placement of a nasogastric or gastrostomy tube is a specific medical intervention, not a normal aspect of feeding. We agree and believe that the choice *not* to use a feeding tube should be explicitly offered.

Is the placement of a feeding tube *desirable?* There is no single answer to this question (see Chapter 11). Feeding through tubes can provide balanced nutrition, thereby improving the body's function and prolonging life. However, feeding through a tube deprives a person of the pleasure and dignity of eating "naturally" and can lead to aspiration of food into the lungs. Being fed through a tube also deprives a person of the communal/sharing aspects of feeding.

We also believe that a feeding tube can be removed at any time just as medical treatment can be stopped. Some individuals would disagree with these ideas and contend that, since the individual is being starved, removal of a tube is always ethically inappropriate. Our opinion that feeding via a tube is a medical treatment is supported by the recognition that there are significant side effects of artificial feeding.

Because most patients who are unable to eat or seem to refuse to eat are usually severely demented, they are almost never able to participate in a clear, consistent, and reasoned discussion about death, suicide, or refusing to eat. We believe it unlikely that most individuals in this circumstance are *choosing* not to eat. Their severe cognitive impairment prevents them from appreciating the complexities of their circumstances. It seems particularly inappropriate to *assume* that food refusal results from a person's realization of the severity of their condition without their telling us. We believe it is inappropriate to *guess* that not eating is a choice of the ill person without being told this directly and repeatedly by them. Because depression is difficult to diagnose in patients with dementia, is potentially treatable, and is a cause of life-threatening food refusal, treatment for depression should be attempted if the possibility exists that it underlies food refusal.

If families are considering not placing a feeding tube in a person who resides in a nursing home, we urge them to discuss this directly with the staff and administration. Some homes are unwilling to let a person starve to death but an increasing number see the placement of a tube in the patient as invasive and one that the patient or family can choose or reject. If chosen, a decision to remove the tube can be made in the future. Experience tells us, however, that the decision to remove a tube is very difficult emotionally.

One question that sometimes arises is whether starvation causes pain to the patient. This is impossible to answer with complete confidence. However, based on the reports of individuals who recover from severe dehydration and who report that they were not uncomfortable, we believe it very unlikely that this is a painful or uncomfortable state. Furthermore, patients who do not eat appear to be comfortable and do not complain of hunger. Thus, when caregivers ask about discomfort we discuss our conclusion that it is unlikely.

The question of what to do for individuals with no available family, no legal guardian, and no well-documented evidence about prior desires is less difficult. While some argue that a third party—for example, a court-appointed guardian or ombudsman—should make a decision based on an "educated guess" or quality-of-life assessment of what this person might have wanted, we believe this is inappropriate. Since the sanctity of human life requires that professionals act to preserve life unless a fully competent person chooses otherwise, in the absence of a person who is aware of the prior wishes of the ill person or the family's own wishes, professionals and society should act to support life.

There is no single right answer to the questions surrounding feeding tube placement. The patient's prior wishes have primary weight and should guide treatment. The professional should provide information and emotional support, raise questions, encourage discussion, and allow time for a decision to develop. Not feeding is an emotionally difficult option but it can be ethically appropriate.

LEGAL ISSUES

Determining Capacity or Competency

In the United States, adults have the legal right to make all decisions for themselves and their children. *Competency,* the ability to make decisions, is automatically established when a person reaches the age of adulthood. It is a legal concept. *Incompetency* is a legal concept that refers to a decision made by a judge that a person lacks the ability to make responsible decisions.

The term *capacity* refers to the abilities a person needs to make decisions. It is a clinical concept. Intact capacity requires three capacities: (1) the ability to communicate, (2) the ability to understand what is being communicated, and (3) the ability to make decisions. Incapacity implies impairments in one of these plus a diagnosable condition that is causing these impairments.

In the past, capacity has been considered either present or absent. It is now recognized that a capacity can be partially present. The majority of those who have impaired decision-making capacity have the capacity to make some decisions but not others. Only the most severely cognitively impaired lack the capacity to express *any* opinions about their desires and make choices. For example, patients who cannot live independently or prepare meals can express preference for clothing, choose if they would like to go on a trip, or ask for a specific food. That is, different *levels* of capacity are required in different circumstances. Therefore, the clinician assessing capacity must examine both the person's abilities to comprehend and decide *and* the potential outcomes of a decision. If serious harm is likely, a greater burden is placed on the patient to demonstrate capacity. When harm is unlikely or nonexistent there is little reason to invoke incompetency.

The inability to precisely define terms like capacity and competency is sometimes a source of frustration among clinicians. Complicating the matter further is the fact that decision-making capacity can change over time. Some medical conditions that impair decision-making capacity (for example, delirium) are reversible. Thus, a person who suffers from a permanent dementia may undergo a sudden decline in capacity due to a urinary tract infection and then regain capacity after treatment.

This potential variability in capacity has several implications. First, if there is some potential for improvement in the patient's condition and a decision in question does not need to be made immediately, it is better to delay an opinion on decision-making capacity as long as possible. Even when an immediate decision must be made, repeat examinations over several hours may elicit periods of lucidity and retained decision-making capacity. This could provide information about the patient's desires in a specific instance.

Furthermore, the concepts of capacity and competency have strong components of cultural shaping. Therefore, it is likely that their definitions will change over time and will vary among different cultures and legal jurisdictions.

The following paragraphs list six issues the clinician can review when assessing whether a person with dementia has intact decision-making capacity. They are also listed in Table 12.1. In the end, the clinician must make a clinical judgment based on the available information. Elements 1–3 assess whether the person can understand the issue at hand. Elements 4–6 assess whether the person can assess the options and make a choice. If the person is able to meet all six elements, their capacity is intact. If they meet one but not all the criteria, they are partially impaired but still may have adequate capacity for some decisions. When the capacity to decide is partially intact, the assessment of whether a person has the capacity to make a particular decision depends on the potential risks and benefits of that decision.

1. *Identify the issue at hand*? As a starting point, the patient should be able to state what the issue is. A capable person will be able to verbally repeat and summarize the question. Individuals who are unable to verbally communicate may be able to do so in a written fashion. In persons with severe language disorders, four or five options can be provided. If the person consistently chooses the issue at hand, then this criterion would be satisfied.

This criterion is aimed at assuring that all parties are discussing the same issue. It does not assess whether the person "understands." Several other criteria below are attempts to operationalize the capacity to "understand." Examples of meeting a criterion would be statements such as, "The doctor says I need an operation" or "The social worker doesn't think I can live by myself."

Table 12.1. Six Elements to Deciding Capacity in Dementia Patients

Can the dementia patient
1. Identify the issue at hand?
2. State the major options to address the issue?
3. Know the most likely outcome(s) of each option?
4. State a choice from among the options?
5. Provide a reason that justifies the choice?
6. Show consistency over time?

2. Can the person state the major options? If the person is able to list the major options or possible decisions, this demonstrates that he or she has the appreciation that a choice among options must be made.

3. Can the person state the most likely outcome or outcomes of each major option? The level of sophistication of this discussion might vary widely depending on the patient's innate ability and willingness to cooperate. Statements such as "The doctor says I'll probably die if I don't get this operation" or "I know I could freeze to death if I sleep here" demonstrate a knowledge of potential outcome and support the conclusion that the patient has the capacity to comprehend the question at hand.

4. Does the person state a choice from among the options? A key element of capacity determination is assessing whether the individual has the capacity to make decisions. The demonstration that a choice has been made is central to this. Affirmative responses to the first three elements address the patient's ability to consider the specific question being discussed. This criterion establishes whether the person is expressing a specific choice.

5. Does the person give a "reason" that justifies their choice? This is positive evidence that a decision is being made. However, the inability or refusal to give a reason cannot be used as the sole basis for deciding that a person lacks capacity. Statements such as, "Because that's what I want" offer no evidence.

Requiring a "rational" reason imposes too strict a standard and would limit a person's ability to make an unusual or uncommon decision. Reasons that derive from delusions, misperceptions that cannot be corrected, or repeated misunderstanding and misstatements of "facts" are evidence that a person lacks ability. However, a person's willingness to state reasons should be considered positive evidence that decision-making capacity is intact.

6. Is the person consistent over time? The person who consistently repeats the same decision is offering evidence that a choice has been made. Obviously, people must have the ability to change their opinions. Indecision or changing a decision is not abnormal, but when the capacity of a person to make decisions is in question and the person is constantly changing, it is appropriate to question his decision-making capacity. The ability to give reasons for changing a decision should increase the clinician's confidence that the individual has altered a choice—that is, has made another choice. Refusal to give reasons for a change or apparent inability to do so cannot, in itself, be used as evidence that a person lacks capacity.

If a given patient does not have the capacity to decide, the clinician must look to see if a psychiatric or medical disorder is present which "explains" the incapacity. Clinicians are empowered by the courts to give expert testimony about capacity because of their ability to identify medical and psychiatric conditions that have caused the incapacity. Dementia, mental retardation, delusional depression, and schizophrenia are *potential* causes of impaired capacity. The mere presence of any one of these disorders, however, is not evidence that a person is incapable of making decisions. Medical testimony is necessary to link the impairments in understanding, reasoning, and choosing (Table 12.1) to the conclusion that the person lacks the capacity to make decisions.

Testamentary Capacity

Testamentary capacity is the ability to write a will. In most jurisdictions three abilities are necessary for intact testamentary capacity: (1) knowledge of assets, (2) knowledge of how assets are "usually" distributed, and (3) an explicit statement of how (and perhaps why) the person is choosing to distribute assets.

As can be seen, these are much more specific criteria than in the previous paragraphs. One reason is that will writing is a very specific ability. Another is that will-making has a long tradition of importance, so case law has developed. Finally, leaving possessions to one's heirs has important links to family values. Criteria for overturning a will are very strict. Thus, a person can be impaired in many areas of function and yet be fully able to prepare or change a will. Since a will can be contested, we suggest a specific assessment of the three issues listed in the paragraph if a person with dementia wishes to draw up or change a will.

Durable Powers of Attorney

Power of attorney is a legal term that refers to the delegation of legal powers. It usually delegates to another person (the *attorney*) the ability (*power*) to sign papers or carry out other legal processes. Because it is a delegation of a legal right, a person must be competent to delegate power of attorney. In addition a person must remain competent for the power of attorney to be enforced since the individual has the right to remove or discontinue the power of attorney at any time.

Because dementing illnesses often interfere with a person's capacity and often lead to incompetency many states have implemented a *durable power of attorney*. This is usually worded such that it persists even after a person becomes incompetent. It may be worded so that it only begins at the time incompetency develops or it may begin while a person is still competent and then continue if they lose this capacity.

In some jurisdictions the durable power of attorney is divided into several types. A common distinction is made between durable power of attorney for health matters and for financial matters. Health matters relate to agreeing to medical care, signing for operations, and making life-and-death decisions. Financial matters usually relate to buying and selling property and other monetary issues.

We recommend that all dementia patients set up a durable power of attorney meeting the laws in their state. This should be done as early as possible so as to prevent any questions about a patient's capacity to appoint an "attorney." This also allows patients to decide ahead of time who will manage their affairs and also avoids the necessity of having a judge assign a guardian.

Advance Directives

In the past decade many jurisdictions in the United States have set up legal documents by which an individual can direct others to make future health decisions for them if they become unable to do so themselves. The first such document was the *Living Will*. This states a person's wishes if he or she becomes terminally ill. In fact, decisions about terminal care are a small part of health care decisions. A new document, called *Advance Directives*, was then developed and is available in almost all states. This allows competent individuals to designate who should make health decisions for them if they become incapacitated. It also allows a person to state wishes about such matters as the use of feeding tubes, ventilators, and aggressive treatment at the end of life.

We see little use for the Living Will as it is too narrow, too flexible, and only covers decision making in terminal phases of an illness. However, the Advance Directives is an important document and we encourage all our patients who have the capacity to draw one up to do so.

Living Wills

A living will is a document in which wishes about medical care at the end of life can be stated. In order for it to become effective, the person must be declared terminally ill—that is, close to death. Therefore, we see little benefit in having a Living Will. It is difficult to know ahead of time what medical decisions will need to be made. Furthermore, terminal care covers a short period of time and the most difficult decisions usually arise before a person is terminally ill. We recommend this durable power of attorney as a better method of ensuring that one's wishes will be followed.

GENERAL CONCLUSIONS AND PRINCIPLES

Several principles can be derived from the above discussions. Attempts should be made to maximize the independence and self-determination of persons with dementia. While dementia often limits an individual's judgment and decision-making capacity, many persons with dementia have retained capacity to decide some or all issues that control their health care. Attempts should be made to preserve whatever ability is retained.

Some dilemmas can be avoided by "preventive" ethics. Early discussion can avoid the need for rushed, last-minute discussions. All individuals should be encouraged to discuss with others their preferences regarding life support, surgery, and other significant interventions while they have the capacity to do so. All individuals should be urged to appoint a *durable power of attorney for health matters* who will be legally empowered to make decisions for them if they become disabled. Ideally, this will be done long before health problems develop.

A diagnosis of dementia in no way limits access to adequate medical, social, and psychological care. Most mildly impaired individuals have the capacity to discuss, decide, and express their wishes. The presence of severe deficits should be taken as an indication that care must be carefully supervised and supported since the person is not able to defend him or herself.

Substituted judgment is best supplied by a person chosen by the sick person before they become incapacitated. Often this will be a family member, but not always. A legal opinion should be sought only when the durable power of attorney has been designated when no family is available, when there is significant disagreement among available family, or when the family's or surrogate's self-interests appear to be affecting their choice of what is in the patient's best interest.

Most ethical dilemmas are solved by discussion. The clarification of medical, social, and financial issues; the expression of feelings; and an exploration of practical solutions almost always lead the interested parties to agree on an ethically acceptable course of action. *Consensus building* is an effective and attainable method of resolution. After the "medical facts" have been discussed, the potential options and their consequences should be reviewed. Choices can often be narrowed in this way and the discussion focused on specific questions and information.

Grief, anger, and guilt should be raised as issues if present. Airing these feelings openly can help clarify sources of disagreement. They are powerful shapers of the decision-making process. Their expression and clarification can allow the decision making to proceed.

Clinical Genetics
and Dementia

*I*n almost all human diseases, there is an interaction between nature and nurture. For some diseases, such as Huntington disease, inheritance determines whether the disease will occur, while the environment may influence its age of onset, clinical presentation and severity. Other diseases—for example, head trauma or toxin exposure—are caused by environmental factors but modified in clinical expression by genetic factors. In Alzheimer disease, multiple genes are involved; some cause the disease and others modify (increasing or decreasing) the likelihood of its occurring or affect the age at which symptoms develop.

Our understanding of the clinical genetics of the dementias is in its infancy, but clinicians caring for patients with dementia should still have a basic understanding of genetics. Knowledge of genetic contributions to the cause and expression of dementia will increasingly influence treatment in the future. In addition, understanding the pattern of inheritance will help the clinician provide genetic counseling or help the clinician know when to refer to a genetic counselor. Relatives, particularly offspring, of those afflicted with dementia may then understand their own personal risk for the disease as well as the risk of their offspring.

This chapter first outlines basic genetic principles. Genetic testing and counseling is then discussed to set the context for the genetic counseling of persons related to patients with dementia. In particular, we discuss presymptomatic testing, genetic counseling, and estimating risk. Finally, we briefly apply knowledge gained from genetics to the care of patients with three diseases, Alzheimer disease, Huntington disease, and vascular dementia.

A GENETICS PRIMER

Chromosomes are complex molecules made up of deoxyribonucleic acid (DNA) that involve a variety of other proteins. They are carried in the nucleus of cells and have a very dense central point (centromere), from which a long arm (q arm) and a short arm (p arm) emanate. Each human cell carries a total of 46 chromosomes, all of which are in pairs. Chromosomes 1–22 are referred to as the autosomal chromosomes. There are two copies of each. Humans also carry two sex chromosomes: Women have two copies of the X chromosome and men one copy of the X and one copy of the Y.

Genes are made up of long strings of DNA contained on chromosomes. Each human has roughly 100,000 genes. (The actual number has yet to be determined.) Each gene codes for a distinct protein. Proteins are the basic structural and functional foundation of the body.

Since there are two copies of each chromosome, there are two copies of every gene, each of which is referred to as an allele. Because a copy of each gene comes from each parent, the two alleles are not always identical. This allows for redundancy, so if we carry one aberrant gene, a second normal gene coding for the same protein may allow us to function as humans. The variation in amino acid sequence of a gene is called a *polymorphism*.

During reproduction each parent produces either sperm or ova, which contain half their own genetic material. Thus a father contributes into his sperm one copy of chromosome 1, one copy of chromosome 2, and so on. Half his sperm contain a Y chromosome and the other half contain an X chromosome. The assortment of different chromosomes (and therefore genes) in individual sperm cells is random, allowing for a tremendous amount of variation. Similarly, the mother places in her ovum (egg) through the process known as *meiosis* one-half of her genetic material. When the sperm fertilizes the egg the new human organism has a full complement of chromosomes (half from each parent). Because of this process of reproduction, individual genes are inherited as separate particles, independent of one another. Parental characteristics do not blend in offspring but are rather present in offspring as an aggregate of individual parts.

Genes vary in function, so it follows that specific diseases are associated with particular genes. Aberrancies in some genes do not allow viability of the fetus and account for the relatively high rate of undetected spontaneous miscarriages. In some instances it is possible to live a normal life with only one functioning gene. Under biologic stress, however, having only one functioning gene may result in transient symptoms of a disease that resolve when the stress resolves. Aberrant genes may code for aberrant proteins that cause malregulation of other genes and lead to the expression of a disease in all those who carry it.

Several distinct inheritance patterns of disease have been described. In the *autosomal patterns,* a defective gene is carried on one of the 22 nonsex chromosomes and is the cause of disease. If a single copy of the aberrant gene is sufficient to produce the disease, this is referred to as the *autosomal dominant* situation. A disease inherited autosomal dominantly occurs in every successive generation and afflicts, on average, one-half of the offspring. Huntington disease is an example of this. Looking carefully at the pedigree (a genetic diagram) of an individual with dementia can help us appreciate whether the disease is being transmitted autosomal dominantly.

In *autosomal recessive* inheritance, two copies of an aberrant gene are necessary to express the disease. In this way the gene may be carried down several generations and remain silent because the offspring do not mate with individuals who also carry the aberrant gene. This is referred to as a *carrier state.* Occasionally there will be a chance pairing between two carriers of the gene, which results in the development of the disease in approximately one-fourth of their offspring—that is, in those who inherit two aberrant genes, one from each of their two healthy parents. Cystic fibrosis is an example of autosomal recessive inheritance.

The third general pattern of inheritance is referred to as *sex-linked.* If the abnormal gene is carried on an X chromosome, it behaves like a recessive in women, who carry only one affected X chromosome. However, in men who only have one X chromosome, the disease will act as a dominant and will occur in every male who inherits the aberrant X chromosome. As a result, sex-linked disease occurs almost exclusively in males of a particular family and skips generations if there are no male offspring. Hemophilia is an example of X-linked inheritance.

The final general category of inherited diseases is known as *multifactorial.* In this paradigm several genes must be aberrant at the same time for a disease to develop. Inheritance is neither dominant nor recessive and several generations may be skipped before it is expressed. Most of the common dementias have multifactorial inheritance.

A variety of genetic tests are available and more are being developed. The simplest is a direct examination of the chromosome and is referred to as *karyotyping.* It involves drawing blood and examining peripheral white blood cells (lymphocytes) after chemical fixation of the cell in the nuclei. Under the microscope or by photographic enlargement the general appearance of the chromosomes can be examined and gross aberrancies such as large pieces of missing or duplicated chromosomes can be identified. Trisomy 21 (Down syndrome) is diagnosed in this fashion. Currently, most of the chromosomal conditions are diagnosed by karyotyping.

Other tests involve looking specifically at the DNA by drawing blood or taking dead cell samples by gently scraping the mouth cavity. The simplest test is restriction fragment length polymorphism (RFLP). It has been known for some time that if certain enzymes are added to DNA solutions they cut the DNA at predetermined sites. DNA in the form of "DNA soup" can then be studied to look at the fragments left after cuts with different restriction enzymes. This process allows the creation of large libraries that document what happens to normal DNA after it is cut with specific restriction enzymes. It then becomes possible to predict the lengths that different parts of DNA will be cut into when it is normal and cut with specific enzymes. Taking DNA from persons with different diseases and applying different restriction enzymes can lead to finding DNA of different lengths (and therefore different molecular composition) because of a difference in sequence. Systematic comparisons of different lengths allow scientists to identify which segments of DNA may be involved in particular diseases. More elaborate tests then allow us to look at specific segments and regions of DNA and eventually allow the identification of specific genes involved in different diseases.

It is also possible to test for the presence or absence of aberrant genes for thousands of diseases in the human genome. In the future it will be possible to test individuals for the presence or absence of individual aberrant genes in their genetic makeup even in the absence of disease. This will be done simply by drawing blood from the individual involved. Already this is possible with Huntington disease, because the gene for the condition has been identified on the short arm of chromosome 4. Individuals at risk for this disease can now be tested and be told with 100% certainty whether they will develop the disease or not. What they cannot be told is when it will develop or exactly what the symptoms will be.

These advances in genetics diagnosis have led us into a new era. They raise many problems as well as many possibilities. The experience at Johns Hopkins with presymptomatic testing for Huntington disease has been that the majority of individuals at risk for Huntington disease are not interested in finding out whether or not they carry the diseased gene. With the proper approach, genetic counseling of those who *are* interested evolves smoothly. Genetic counseling and presymptomatic testing related to dementia are likely to become widespread in the years to come.

GENETIC COUNSELING AND PRE-SYMPTOMATIC TESTING IN DEMENTIA

Genetic counseling communicates information about the genetic aspects of dementia and provides support to relatives of persons with dementia. Genetic counselors are health care professionals who are trained in the technical and clinical aspects of a genetic disease. However, certain groups of health care professionals such as physicians or psychologists may also be qualified to provide genetic counseling. The purpose of the counseling is twofold. The first is to provide general information about the heritability of particular dementing disorders. This basically involves the communication of knowledge that has been acquired through research. Second, genetic counseling is intended to provide specific advice to relatives, typically children, of persons with dementia regarding their own risk of developing dementia.

Several steps are involved in genetic counseling: obtaining a complete history and pedigree, conducting an examination of the affected individual, ordering appropriate laboratory investigations, and the act of counseling itself. As applied to dementia, genetic counseling involves the determination of a phenotype of the patient's dementia using the evaluation practices in Chapter 2. When possible, the specific etiology of the dementia should be identified—that is Alzheimer disease, vascular dementia, Huntington disease, and so on. Pathologic diagnosis of the cause of dementia is important although not always available. Finally, genotyping of the affected individual with respect to abnormal genes is conducted.

Perhaps the most important aspect of genetic counseling involves gaining an understanding of the individuals who are seeking it. A clear delineation of their motives for requesting genetic counseling is the first subject that needs to be addressed. Are they interested in learning whether they might develop the disease so that they can prepare psychologically? Are they thinking of having children and therefore want to know whether they are carrying an aberrant gene that would put their children at risk? Or is there some other reason, perhaps a financial motive, that might be involved?

Another aspect of genetic counseling is an assessment of the psychological impact of test results. Are individuals at high risk of severe emotional upset if the results are distressing? Are there people close to them such as family members or friends who would support them if they have inherited the disease gene? Would they be amenable to long-term counseling to help them emotionally if they become significantly upset or depressed?

Finally, genetic counseling helps people consider what they are likely to do with the information and how it might affect their lives. In the past, concerns have been raised about bad news leading people to suicide. Experience with the Baltimore Huntington Disease Presymptomatic Testing Project at Johns Hopkins suggests that this almost never happens, but suicidal ideation and severe depression are potential risks. Those being counseled are specifically asked to consider how they would anticipate reacting if they were told that they are carrying a gene that puts them at serious risk for developing a very bad disease. Thorough, careful consideration of this question is crucial before genetic testing is undertaken.

Genetic testing of individuals with a family history of dementia is currently most informative for the uncommon families in which a dominant mode of inheritance is present. The population rate of dementia is so high that it is not possible with the present state of knowledge to estimate precisely the risk of dementia in most people with a relative who has dementia.

What can be said with certainty for most cases of dementia is that the relatives of people with dementia are at higher risk for developing dementia than the general population and that this risk increases with age. How much greater this risk is cannot be stated with precision except for a few relatively uncommon diseases. One study has suggested that the first degree relative (parent, sibling, child) of a person with Alzheimer disease has a 38% chance of developing Alzheimer in their lifetime.

As our understanding of the human genome increases and our ability to link specific genotypes to specific dementing disorders improves, it will be possible to give individuals more precise estimates of their genetic risk. Given the experience of the Baltimore Huntington Disease Presymptomatic Testing Project, in which few first degree relatives of persons with Huntington disease were interested in finding out their own genetic risk, we anticipate that this information will be useful to some individuals. However, most will not seek testing until effective interventions or preventive treatments are available. Some of these issues will be discussed further in reviewing the genetics of three diseases associated with dementia.

Alzheimer Disease

Alzheimer disease with onset before age 60 is often of a genetic etiology, transmitted as autosomal dominantly, and caused by genetic abnormalities on chromosomes 1, 14, 21 and others that are not yet known. The observation that almost 100% of people with Down syndrome develop the pathology of AD by age 40 led to an investigation of chromosome 21 since there is either an extra chromosome 21 or an extra piece of this chromosome in people with Down syndrome. The gene that directs the production of the amyloid precursor protein (APP—see Chapter 3) is involved in the production of amyloid plaque found in Alzheimer, and is found on chromosome 21. Several different mutations in this gene result in an abnormal form of this protein being produced and lead to the development of Alzheimer disease. This overproduction of the amyloid precursor protein is also likely involved in the association of Alzheimer disease and Down syndrome. The presenilin-1 gene on chromosome 14 and the presenilin-2 gene on chromosome 1 produce proteins whose function is poorly known but probably involve the metabolism of APP.

A different mode of action is associated with the apolipoprotein E gene (APOE), which is located on chromosome 19. This gene has three alleles, labeled 2, 3, and 4. Carrying allele 4 (APOE-ε4) places people at risk for developing Alzheimer disease at a younger age. The gene product does not appear to cause the disease directly. Rather, it seems to modify its age of onset. Individuals who carry two ε4 alleles have an earlier age of onset than individuals with one ε4 allele, but several people in their 90s have been identified who have two ε4 alleles but do not suffer from Alzheimer disease.

More recently, it has been reported that an abnormal form of the chromosome 12 gene coding for alpha-2 macroglobulin (alpha-2M) is also a strong risk factor for the onset of Alzheimer disease in later life. As many as 30% of the population carry the mutation. It is still not known precisely how this abnormal gene increases the risk for AD, although it appears that alpha-2M is involved in the clearance of amyloid from brain tissue. This finding must be replicated before being accepted.

Given the issues reviewed above, we suggest the following. First, it is crucial to conduct a careful evaluation to confirm the diagnosis of Alzheimer disease in affected relatives, if possible, through pathologic investigation of the affected relative. Second, genetic testing of patients and relatives should be considered only when there is a clear genetic pattern in the pedigree such as autosomal dominant transmission with early onset disease. In very rare cases, interested relatives, particularly children, might undergo genetic testing to determine whether or not they possess one of the abnormal genes on chromosome 1, 14, or 21. At present, genetic testing for apolipoprotein ε4 and alpha-2M polymorphisms is *not* appropriate for relatives of patients with suspected Alzheimer disease.

In the near future other genes will be identified that increase or decrease the risk of developing Alzheimer disease. At present, genetic testing is appropriate for only a minority of cases of patients and relatives, since the majority of Alzheimer patients are late onset and most do not have a family history. In the future, combinations of genetic testing, brain imaging, and detailed neuropsychological testing may predict whether individuals are at risk for developing Alzheimer disease and what their likelihood is of developing symptoms by a specific age.

Huntington Disease

From its earliest descriptions, Huntington disease has been recognized as a genetic disorder. In affected families it occurs in every generation, and it afflicts approximately half of each successive generation in an autosomal dominant pattern. In 1984 the disease was linked to a gene on chromosome 4 and in 1993 the aberrant gene was identified. It is now possible to diagnose persons at risk for Huntington disease genetically and to determine with near 100% certainty whether or not they will develop the disease if they live long enough.

The genetic abnormality causing Huntington disease is an increased number of repeat amino acid sequences in a gene that produces a protein called *huntingtin*. Normal people have a string of fewer than 30–32 repeats, called *triplet repeats* of three amino acids (cytosine, adenosine, guanine—CAG). Patients with Huntington disease have 37 or more of these repeats. The more triplet repeats a person has, the earlier the age of onset of the disease. Additionally when the disease is transmitted through a male proband—that is, from father to child—there are usually more triplet repeats in the child's genome than in the father's. This process, in which a genetic defect grows worse as it passes down the generations, is referred to as *anticipation*. By taking a simple blood test and determining the number of CAG triplet repeats in the HD gene, it is possible to determine whether or not a person will develop the disease with 100% certainty. Thus, genetic counseling is particularly applicable to Huntington disease because of the high degree of certainty provided by the testing. Nevertheless, the experience at Johns Hopkins is that less than half of those at risk for Huntington disease are interested in finding out whether or not they carry the aberrant gene.

Vascular Dementia

The genetics of vascular dementia are poorly understood. There is evidence that a family history of dementia is more prevalent in patients with vascular dementia than it is in the general population. This suggests a role for genetics in the development of vascular dementia. However, this role remains unclear. One possible explanation involves the observation that many cases diagnosed clinically with vascular dementia turn out to also have Alzheimer disease. Therefore, it may be that this genetic association involves that subcategory of cases with comorbid Alzheimer and vascular dementia.

Another possible explanation is that the genetic association is a linkage of risk factors for stroke. Diabetes, hypertension, and high cholesterol, all conditions with genetic associations, increase the risk for stroke; familial association may be due to the increased risk for diabetes, hypercholesterolemia, and hypertension in relatives of stroke patients. A final possible explanation is that certain types of vascular dementia have specific genetic components.

At this point it is extremely difficult to disentangle these three possibilities without further evidence. Thus genetic counseling for patients who have vascular dementia is not currently practical.

Glossary

affect: the outward expression of individuals' subjective of emotional state as manifested in their behavior. Important elements of affect include range, changeability, and rapidity of change.

aggression: a verbal or physical act which produces harm or carries the potential of harm to self, an individual, or object. Examples of aggression in dementia include screaming, the use of profanity, and specific behaviors such as hitting, kicking, spitting, biting, and pushing.

agnosia: a disturbance of perception in which the ability to recognize or interpret primary perceptions is impaired. Agnosia impairs the ability to interpret perceptions in all the senses: vision, hearing, touch, smell, and taste. For example, an individual may be able to see a face and recognize and name the parts of the face but not know that this face belongs to a specific familiar person (prosopagnosia). Another common example is a person whose left side is paralyzed but is totally unaware of this (nosagnosia) and denies it even when shown the paralyzed limbs.

akathisia: a subjective state of restlessness, sometimes described as the urge to jump out of one's skin. This may manifest itself in the person's being in constant motion, pacing, switching weight from one leg to another when standing, stamping feet, or crossing and uncrossing legs when sitting. This is a side effect of antipsychotic medication or a consequence of certain neurologic diseases.

amnesia: a primary disturbance of memory which manifests itself as a loss of memory for previously learned events (retrograde amnesia) or an inability to learn new material (anterograde amnesia.)

amnestic disorder: a cognitive disorder in which memory impairment is the only abnormality. The most common form of amnestic syndrome is Korsakoff's syndrome, which is associated with damage to the thalamus or mammillary bodies.

anosoagnosia (see also agnosia): lack of awareness of a deficit.

antipsychotic medications: a type of medication typically used to treat delusions, hallucinations, or thought disorder but also used to treat aggression and other behavioral disturbances in dementia. These medications are sometimes called *neuroleptics* because of their neurologic side effects, including parkinsonism, akathisia, dystonia, tardive dyskinesia, and neuroleptic malignant syndrome. Examples include haloperidol (Haldol), risperidone (Risperdal), olanzapine (Zyprexa), thioridazine (Mellaril), and others (see Chapter 10).

antidepressants: medications from different chemical classes which reduce depressive symptoms in patients with mood disorder. Four classes are distinguished: tricyclic antidepressants, selective serotonin reuptake inhibitors, monoamine oxidase inhibitors, and newer antidepressants.

antidepressants, newer: newer classes of antidepressant medicines which appear to have milder side effects. They come from several chemical classes and have been broadly used in dementia. Examples include bupropion (Wellbutrin), venlafaxine (Effexor), trazodone (Desyrel), nefazodone (Serzone), and mertazapine (Remeron).

anxiety: a mental symptom characterized by apprehension, tension, uneasiness, and/or worry.

anxiety disorder: a syndrome of sustained anxiety with accompanying physical symptoms (muscle tension, tremor, rapid heartbeat) that may involve panic attacks, obsessions, or compulsions.

apathy: a state of reduced interest and initiative.

aphasia: a disturbance of language manifested as difficulties in communicating. Aphasic individuals may have trouble *understanding* spoken or written language (receptive aphasia, fluent aphasia, Wernicke's aphasia), repeating spoken language (communicating aphasia), or *expressing* themselves in verbal or written language (expressive aphasia, nonfluent aphasia, Broca's aphasia). In *transcortical* aphasia, repetition is intact but there is difficulty with either understanding or expression or both.

apraxia: the inability to carry out a learned, complex motor task in the absence of paralysis or movement difficulty (such as with Parkinson disease.) Common motor tasks affected by apraxia in dementia include dressing, grooming, driving, and eating.

ataxia: a disturbance in gait in which patients have trouble coordinating the movements involved in walking. Ataxic gaits may be broadbased, "magnetic" (the person's feet stick to the ground and are slow to lift and move around), and unstable.

athetosis: a sustained, writhing movement of limbs, trunk, or neck which is involuntary.

atrophy: a loss of tissue in the body. Muscle tissue atrophy occurs after the development of paralysis in the muscles which are no longer used. In dementia, atrophy of the brain is seen when brain tissue is lost.

behavior disorder: an observable activity of an individual that is disruptive or dangerous or is associated with distress in the patient or those around the patient.

behavioral perspective: the logic of attributing a mental or behavioral disturbance to a disturbance of one of the innate drives (sleep, eating, sexuality) or to the "taking over" of the individual's behavior by a single maladaptive cycle of behavior with a specific goal (for example, to be seen as sick, to restrict eating, or to abuse alcohol). The behavior perspective focuses attention on observable behaviors and the rules that govern them such as reward and punishment.

benzodiazepines: a class of medications which have activity at a specific receptor site in the brain (the benzodiazepine receptor site) of the GABA system. Typically, these medications have sedating and anxiolytic (anxiety relieving) properties. Chronic use can lead to addiction. Their use in brain injured individuals, including patients with dementia, can lead to disinhibition. Examples include diazepam (Valium), chlordiazepoxide (Librium), oxazepam (Serax), lorazepam (Ativan), and clonazepam (Klonopin).

catastrophic reaction: a sudden, extreme emotional, physical, or behavioral response to a seemingly minor stimulus as if it were a catastrophe.

catatonia: a clinical syndrome characterized by near immobility of movement and thought, punctuated by shorter periods of excitability and overactivity. Catatonic patients are mute, move very little, and may exhibit "waxy flexibility" (moving their limbs feels to an examiner as if they are being moved through wax).

chorea: a dance-like, rapid, involuntary movement of the limbs, trunk or neck, seen in Huntington disease.

circumlocutory language (see also aphasia): a style of language in which an individual appears to use a series of phrases in the place of more precise individual words. For example, "hand me the writing instrument while I am preparing to inscribe what I'm trying to say."

cognition: the sum total of human thinking, reasoning, and abstracting capacities.

cognitive disorder, mild: a condition in which there are impairments in several areas of cognition, but not severe enough to be a dementia or to affect functioning.

cogwheeling: a neurologic sign elicited by an examiner's moving an individual's limb or muscle group back and forth. It consists of intermittent "catching" followed by relaxation of a muscle, similar to how the cogs of a wheel catch and release.

compulsion (see also obsession): an intrusive, repetitive *action* that cannot be resisted (or leads to discomfort and anxiety if resisted) and which is not perceived as alien by the person (it seems to them that it is their own urge). Compulsions may include repetition of certain trivial acts (checking, counting, tapping) or repetitions of complex actions (brushing teeth in a certain way) or behaviors (washing hands), or may simply be an intrusive repetitive action that is distracting from other mental activities.

confabulation: a fabrication of stories in response to questions. Commonly seen in memory disorders in which patients appear to be filling in gaps in their memory.

cortical dementia: a dementia characterized by aphasia, apraxia, agnosia, and amnesia. Cortical dementias typically are due to damage in the brain in the temporal, parietal, and occipital lobes of the brain. Alzheimer disease is the most common cause of cortical dementia.

decreased level of consciousness: a state of impaired clarity or clouding of awareness of the environment and inability to sustain attention. Terms which describe decreased level of consciousness include "drowsiness," stupor, coma. It may manifest as hyper- or hypovigilance.

delirium: an impairment in the level of consciousness and sensorium. Typically it has an acute onset, a specific general medical cause, and resolves after its primary cause is treated. Delirium is a cognitive disorder with most cognitive functions impaired. Patients might manifest any mental symptom during delirium (including anxiety, depression, delusions, or hallucinations). Patients with delirium can be hypervigilant and active or lethargic and withdrawn.

delusion: a fixed, false, idiosyncratic belief.

dementia: a global decline in cognitive capacity occurring in clear consciousness.

depression: a subjective state of sadness or low mood ("the blues") which may appear as in tearfulness or a sad appearance. See also major depression, minor depression, and dysthymia.

dimensional perspective: the logic of casually attributing a mental or behavioral impairment to a mismatch between the person's personality or cognitive vulnerabilities and current circumstances. Dimensional vulnerabilities refer to universal, continuously graded, individual attributes (for example, intelligence, personality dimensions).

disease perspective: the logic causally attributing a mental or behavioral impairment to a process that has caused a broken part in the brain or the body.

dyskinesia: an abnormal, involuntary movement which involves a muscle or muscle group. Dyskinesias can affect the oral–facial musculature, the hands, legs, and trunk. Dyskinesias are often a medication side effect. Examples include the dyskinesia associated with levo-dopa therapy in Parkinson disease and those that develop after chronic use of neuroleptic medications. Withdrawal dyskinesias may last for days, weeks, or months after discontinuation of a neuroleptic. Withdrawal dyskinesias which last for more than several months after discontinuation of a neuroleptic are referred to as *tardive dyskinesia,* a chronic disfiguring condition.

dysphoria: a state of uncomfortable mood. May be seen in both major depression and mania.

dysthymia: chronic, mild depression typically lasting for years, not severe enough to qualify as a major depression

dystonia: a sustained contraction of a muscle or muscle group that usually results in an abnormal position or posture. Examples include tightening of one side of the neck muscles (torticollis); pulling of the eyes up, down, or to the side (occulogyrie crisis); or leaning of the trunk to one side (Tower of Pisa). Most commonly, dystonia is a side effect of antipsychotic medications (such as haloperidol, risperidone, and others). It also occurs in several brain diseases.

emotional incontinence: a sudden, exaggerated expression of emotion which may or may not occur in response to a stimulus. Examples include pathological laughing and crying when an individual unexpectedly cries or laughs but denies the presence of sad or happy mood. It often occurs when there is damage to subcortical structures such as in pseudobulbar palsy or Parkinson's disease.

euphoria: a state of abnormally elevated mood, usually accompanied by increased confidence in one's abilities. May be manifested by frequent laughing and giggling, or other forms of social disinhibition.

euthymia: a descriptor for normally reactive mood and affect.

executive dysfunction: impairments in the ability to initiate, maintain, or stop a cognitive task or a behavior; to abstract; or to make sound judgments. It may manifest as slowness in thinking, mental inflexibility, social disinhibition, perseveration, poor judgment, or difficulty changing tasks. It is associated with damage to frontosubcortical circuits. It may be associated with frontal release signs (reflexes), such as the grasp, snout, and glabellar reflexes.

extrapyramidal symptomatology (EPS): a set of motor symptoms including dystonia, akathisia, and parkinsonism, attributed to dysfunction of the extrapyramidal motor systems of the brain and spinal cord. In dementia these are either side effects of neuroleptic medications or neurologic symptoms of a disease such as disseminated Lewy body disease or Parkinson disease.

festination: a gait disorder which is initiated by a series of rapid small steps (*marche à petits pas*), which steadily increases in speed, and is difficult for the patient to stop.

frontal-subcortical circuits: neuronal pathways in the brain which join specific areas of the frontal lobes and the basal ganglia in functional units. Damage to frontal-subcortical circuits from any disease is associated with certain types of dementia (subcortical dementia), disturbances of executive function, and disinhibited behavior.

functional impairment: impairments in the ability to carry out routine, everyday activities. Two types are distinguished: impairments of instrumental activities of daily living (IADLs) such as work, household tasks, driving, handling finances, telephone use, and transportation; and impairments in activities of daily living (ADLs) such as dressing, bathing, maintaining continence, feeding, transferring, and mobility.

gait: a medical term for walking.

grasp reflex: a reflex in which patients grab onto things when the underpart of their hand is lightly stroked. This reflex often emerges in advanced dementia and may manifest as grabbing onto clothing, bed rail, or caregivers. These reflex behaviors may be inappropriately interpreted as uncooperativeness, aggression, or resistance to care.

hallucination: a perception without a stimulus. Hallucinations can occur in all senses: visual—seeing things that are not present; auditory—hearing voices or sounds; gustatory—experiencing taste; olfactory and tactile—smelling and feeling sensations on skin.

hydrocephalus: an excess collection of cerebrospinal fluid in the brain which can compress brain tissue and lead to neurologic and mental symptoms.

hypomania: a mild state of mania (see *mania*) which does not lead to social, interpersonal, or functional impairment.

illusion: a misperception of a physical stimulus—for example, seeing a figure in dark curtains at night.

irritability: a subjective state of becoming easily irritated or of having a short fuse. This may manifest in an individual's easily becoming angry, threatening, or hostile.

judgment: the mental process of choosing among a set of actions, behaviors, or values.

lability: the degree of changeability in a person's mood. Labile moods change rapidly in response to minimal environmental stimuli. Examples are becoming rapidly hostile or angry with unexpected sounds, or quickly switching from being calm to being depressed or sad.

life-story perspective: the logic of explaining individuals' mental or behavioral disturbance as being an understandable psychological reaction to their life circumstances. For example, "He is upset because he feels lost," and "He wants to eat because he is unhappy in the nursing home."

major depression: a syndrome consisting of persistent low mood, low vital sense (that is, fatiguability, low energy, insomnia, hypersomnia, anorexia), and low self-attitude (for example, a sense of being a burden, low self-esteem, limited confidence, and "emotional vulnerability"). Major depression may be secondary to a general medical condition (such as a stroke or hypothyroidism) or may be *idiopathic*—that is, of unknown cause.

mania: a syndrome characterized by persistent elevation of mood or irritability, elevation in vital sense (that is, with decreased need for sleep, increased energy, and increased activity), and increase in self-attitude, (that is, overconfidence and grandiosity). Mania may also include flight of ideas, in which patients might subjectively feel that their thoughts are going too fast for them to keep track.

mood stabilizers: medications from different chemical classes which have the ability to stabilize swings of mood. These are typically used as treatments for mania, hypomania, and bipolar disorders. Examples include lithium, carbamazepine (Tegretol), divalproex sodium (Depakote), and gabapentin (Neurontin).

mood: an individual's current pervasive, predominant, emotional state. Examples include depression, anxiety, irritability, and euphoria.

myoclonus: a repetitive, intermittent, jerking movement of a muscle or muscle group.

neuroleptic malignant syndrome (NMS): a syndrome consisting of delirium, stiffness, and fever associated with the use of neuroleptic medications. It can develop on low doses and after short term use of these medicines. It is life threatening.

neurotransmitters: chemical substances used by the nervous system for communication between neurons. Many chemical types of neurotransmitters have been described, including peptides and amines. Neurotransmitter systems disturbed in dementia include those that produce acetylcholine, dopamine, norepinephrine, serotonin, and GABA.

obsession (see also compulsion): an intrusive repetitive *urge* or *thought* that an individual tries to resist but ultimately cannot (or that leads to discomfort and anxiety if resisted) and which is not perceived as alien to the person. (It seems as though it is their own.) Obsessions may drive people to do certain acts (see *compulsion*) or may be intrusive, repetitive thoughts that distract from other mental activities.

orthostatic hypotension: a change in blood pressure and pulse that occurs when an individual goes from a lying position to a standing position (after at least 2 minutes). Drops in systolic or diastolic blood pressure of 20 points or more or increases in pulse of 20 points or more constitute clinically significant orthostatic hypotension. Patients with clinically significant orthostatic hypotension typically complain of dizziness or lightheadedness and are at high risk for falls.

overvalued idea: a strongly held idea or belief which arises out of or is reinforced by an individual's immediate cultural environment. Overvalued ideas preoccupy mental life, drive behavior, and lead individuals to act in specific ways. They differ from delusions in that they are not idiosyncratic and are less fixed. Their content is rarely bizarre. Overvalued ideas can be distinguished from ordinary ideas, beliefs, and attitudes in that they typically lead individuals to behave in ways that are outside cultural norms or in some way dangerous to them.

paranoia: a commonly used term referring to suspiciousness or persecutory beliefs. In the original Greek it refers to a tendency to misinterpret events and people as being hostile and directed against the person.

paratonia: a neurologic sign in which there is increasing muscle tone resistance in response to increasing speed of passive limb movement. Paratonia may manifest itself as resistance to movements by others in advanced dementia and can be misinterpreted as aggression or oppositional behavior.

parkinsonism: a motor disturbance in which patients manifest a characteristic tremor (pill rolling), postural disturbance (stooped trunk posture), rigidity or stiffness, mask-like facial expression, slowness in movement (bradykinesia), impaired balance, festination, reduced arm swing, and en bloc turning.

perseveration: the persistence or frequent repetition of a movement or verbal behavior. Examples include an individual repeating a sound or phrase over and over or repeatedly slapping one's thigh. Perseverations are involuntary and may take on the form of an intrusion or repetition of an earlier phrase, sound, or behavior into a new conversation. Perseveration has been associated with damage to frontal-subcortical circuits.

personality: the pervasive and persistent lifelong set of attributes characteristic of an individual, usually unchanging after early adulthood. In dementia, personality can be changed by brain disease. Personality may also "color" dementia patients' mental life and behavior during the course of their illness.

praxis: the ability to carry out a learned motor intervention in the absence of weakness or movement disorder.

selective serotonin reuptake inhibitors (SSRI) (see also antidepressants): a class of antidepressants whose primary mode of activity is believed to involve inhibition of serotonin reuptake into brain neurons. Example includes fluoxetine (Prozac), sertraline (Zoloft), paroxetine (Paxil), and fluvoxamine (Luvox). (See also *antidepressants*.)

self-attitude: an individual's overall sense of him/herself. Impairments in self-attitude can be positive or negative. Negative self-attitude manifests as reduced confidence, hopelessness, guilt, feeling a burden, worthlessness, and low self-esteem. Elevation in self-attitude manifests as overconfidence, grandiosity, and inflated self-esteem.

self-deprecation: a symptom of impaired self-attitude in which personal worth is underestimated.

sign: an observable abnormality in a patient's behavior, noted on interview, physical examination, or mental status examination. A sign may be noted by a clinician or a caregiver.

subcortical dementia: a dementia characterized by the "the four *Ds*": dysmnesia (disturbance in the processing of memory), dysexecutive (executive disturbance), depletion (loss of interest or motivation), and delay (of movement and thought). Subcortical dementias are typically due to disturbances in frontal-subcortical circuits and may be associated with movement disorder and mood. Parkinson disease and Huntington disease are causes of subcortical dementia.

symptom: a complaint reported by a patient—for example, "My head hurts."

syndrome: a characteristic constellation or pattern of signs and symptoms. Dementia is a syndrome characterized by a global decline in intellectual function occurring in clear consciousness.

tardive dyskinesia: see *dyskinesia.*

tone: the resting "tension" or state of a relaxed muscle or muscle group as felt by an observer. Tone can be diminished (hypotonus), normal, or increased (hypertonus). Examples of abnormal tone are rigidity, cogwheeling, spasticity, and paratonia.

transcortical aphasia: see *aphasia.*

tremor: a repetitive, stereotyped, regular movement of a muscle or muscle group which has the appearance of shaking. Tremors occur either at rest or during an action (intention) such as reaching for a glass of water.

tricyclic antidepressants (see also antidepressants): a class of antidepressants whose basic chemical structure is three rings of carbon molecules. They have activity at several brain neurotransmitter systems. Examples include desipramine (Norpramin), imipramine (Tofranil), and nortriptyline (Pamelor).

vital sense: an individual's subjective sense of pep and energy. Reductions in vital sense manifest as feelings of reduced pep or energy or easy fatiguability. Elevations in vital sense might manifest in feeling energized, activated, and constantly on the go.

References

GENERAL

American Psychiatric Association. Diagnostic and Statistical Manual, 4th ed. Washington, DC, 1994.

American Psychiatric Association. Practice guideline for the treatment of patients with Alzheimer disease and other dementias of later life. Am J Psychiatry 1997; 154:5, Suppl:1–39.

Burns A, Levy R. Dementia. Chapman and Hall Medical: London, 1994.

Cummings JL, Benson DF. Dementia: A Clinical Approach. Butterworth-Heineman: Boston, 1992.

Lishman WA. Organic Psychiatry. Blackwell Scientific: Oxford, 1996.

CHAPTER 1: DEFINITIONS AND OVERVIEW OF THE BOOK

Blessed G, Tomlinson BE, Roth M. The association between quantitative measures of dementia and senile change in the cerebral gray matter of elderly subjects. Br J Psychiatry 1968; 114:797–811.

Erkinjuntti T, Ostbve T, Steenhuis R, Hachinski V. The effect of different diagnostic criteria on the prevalence of dementia. N Engl J Med 1997; 337:1667–1674.

Maurer K, Gerbaldo H. Auguste D and Alzheimer's disease. Lancet 1997; 349: 1546–1549.

McHugh PR, Slavney PR. The Perspectives of Psychiatry. Revised edition. Johns Hopkins University Press: Baltimore, 1998.

CHAPTER 2: THE EVALUATION AND FORMULATION OF DEMENTIA

Alexopoulos GS, Abrams RC, Young RC, Shamoian CA. Cornell scale for depression in dementia. Biol Psychiatry 1988; 23:271–284.

Christensen H, Griffiths K, MacKinnon A, Jacomb P. A quantitative review of cognitive deficits in depression and Alzheimer-type dementia. J Int Neuropsychol Soc 1997; 3:631–651.

Cummings JL, Mega M, Gray K, Rosenberg-Thompson S, Carusi DA, Gornbein J. The Neuropsychiatric Inventory: comprehensive assessment of psychopathology in dementia. Neurology 1994; 44:2308–2314.

Folstein MF, Folstein SE, McHugh PR. "Mini-Mental State": a practical method for grading the cognitive state of patients for the clinician. J Psychiatr Res 1975; 2:189–198.

Iliffe S. Can delays in the recognition of dementia in primary care be avoided? Aging Health 1997; 1(1):7–10.

Lawton P, Brody A. Instrumental Activities of Daily Living (IADL) Scale. Incorporated in the Philadelphia Geriatric Center. Multilevel Assessment Instrument (MAI). Psychopharmacology Bulletin 1988; 24:789–791.

Mayeux R, Saunders AM, Shea S, Mirra S, Evans D, Roses AD, Hyman BT, Crain B, Tange MX, Phelps CH. Utility of the apolipoprotein-E genotype in the diagnosis of Alzheimer's disease. N Engl J Med 1998; 338:506–511.

Rabins PV, Steele CS. A scale to measure impairment in severe dementia and similar conditions. Am J Ger Psychiatry 1996; 4:247–251.

Wilkinson IM, Graham-White J. Psychogeriatric Dependency Rating Scales (PGDRS): a method of assessment for use by nurses. Br J Psychiatry 1980; 137:558–565.

CHAPTER 3: DISEASES CAUSING A CORTICAL PATTERN OF DEMENTIA

Hooten RM, Lyketsos CG. Fronto-temporal dementia: a clinicopathological review of four post-mortem studies. J Neuropsychiatry Clin Neurosci 1996; 8:10–19.

McKeith IG, Fairbairn AF, Perry RH, Thompson P. The clinical diagnosis and misdiagnosis of Senile Dementia of the Lewy Body Type (SDLT). Br J Psychiatry 1994; 165:324–332.

McKeith IG, Perry RH, Fairbairn AF, Perry EK. Operational criteria for SDLT. Psychol Med 1992; 22:911–922.

McKhann G, Drachman D, Folstein MF, Katzman R, Price D, Stadlan Ey. Clinical diagnosis of Alzheimer's disease: report of the National Institute Neurologic and Communicative Disorders and Stroke/Alzheimer's Disease Related Disorders Association workgroup under the auspices of DHHS task force on Alzheimer's disease. Neurol 1984; 34:939–944.

Terry RD, Katzman R, Bick KL. Alzheimer Disease. Raven Press: New York, 1994.

CHAPTER 4: DISEASES TYPICALLY CAUSING SUBCORTICAL OR MIXED PATTERN DEMENTIA

Chabriat H, Vahedi K, Iba-Zizen MT, Joutel A, Nibbio A, Nagy TG, Krebs MO, Julien J, Dubois B, Ducrocq X, Levasseur M, Homeyer P, Mas JL, Lyon-Caen O, Tournier Lasserve E, Bousser MG. Clinical spectrum of CADASIL: a study of 7 families. Lancet 1995; 346:934–938.

Folstein S. Huntington Disease: A Disorder of Families. Johns Hopkins University Press: Baltimore, 1992.

Huber SJ, Cummings JL. Parkinson's Disease: Neurobehavioral Aspects. Oxford Press: New York, 1992.
Price RW, Perry SW. HIV, AIDS, and the Brain: ARNMD, Volume 72. Raven Press: New York, 1994.
Rodriguez M, Siva A, Ward J, Stolp-Smith K, O'Brien P, Kurland L. Impairment, disability and handicap in multiple sclerosis. Neurology 1994; 44:28–33.
Romain GC, Tatemichi TK, Erkinjuntti T, Cummings JL, Masdeu JC, Garcia JH, Amaducci L, Ovgogozo JM, Brun A, Hofman A. Vascular dementia: diagnostic criteria for research studies, report of the NINDS-AIREN international workshop. Neurology 1993; 43:250–259.
Silver JM, Yudofsky SC, Hales RE (Eds). Neuropsychiatry of Traumatic Brain Injury. APPI: Washington, DC, 1994.
Schut LJ. Dementia following stroke. Clin Geriatr Med 1988; 4(4):767–784.
Vanneste J, Augustin PA, Dirven C, Tan WF, Goedhart ZD. Shunting normal pressure hydrocephalus: do the benefits outweigh the risks? Neurol 1992; 42: 54–59.
Wu J-C, Choo K-B, Chen C-M, Chen T-Z, Huo T, Lee S-D. Genotyping of hepatitis D virus by restriction-fragment length polymorphism and relation to outcome of hepatitis D. Lancet 1995; 356:939–920.
Yatsu FM, Grotta JC, Pettigrew LC. Stroke. Edward Arnold: London, 1995.
Costa PT, Williams TF, Sommerfield M. Recognition and initial assessment of Alzheimer's disease and related dementias. Practice guideline No. 19, Rockville, MD: U.S. Department of Health and Human Services, Public Health Service, AHCPR Publication No. 97-0702, November 1996.

CHAPTER 5: OVERVIEW OF DEMENTIA CARE

Mace N, Rabins P. The 36-Hour Day. 3rd ed. Johns Hopkins University Press: Baltimore, 1999.
Volicer L, Fabiszewski KJ, Rheaume YL, Lasch KE. Clinical Management of Alzheimer's Disease. Aspen: Rockville, 1988.

CHAPTER 6: SUPPORTIVE CARE FOR THE PATIENT WITH DEMENTIA

Brody J. Guidance in the care of patients with Alzheimer's disease. The New York Times, Wednesday, November 20th, 1983.
Zgola JM. Doing Things: A Guide to Programming Activities for Persons With Alzheimer's Disease and Related Disorders. Johns Hopkins University Press: Baltimore, 1987.

CHAPTER 7: SUPPORTING THE FAMILY AND THE CARE-PROVIDER

Benbow SM, Marriott A, Morley M, Walsh S. Family therapy and dementia: review and clinical experience. Int J Geriatr Psychiatry 1993; 8:717–725.
Hebert R, Leclerc G, Bravo G, Girouard D, Lefrancois G. Efficacy of a support

group programme for caregivers of demented patients in the community: a randomized controlled trial. Arch Gerontol Geriatr 1994; 18:1–14.

Mittelman MS, Ferris SH, Schulman E, Steinberg G, Levin B. A family intervention to delay nursing home placement of patients with Alzheimer disease. JAMA 1996; 276:1725–1731.

Schulz R, O'Brien AT, Bookwala T, Fleiissner K. Psychiatric and physical morbidity effects of dementia caregiving: prevalence, correlates, and causes. Gerontologist 35:771–791, 1995.

CHAPTER 8: NONCOGNITIVE FUNCTIONAL DISORDERS AND DISTURBANCES OF SLEEPING, EATING, AND SEXUALITY

Burns A, Jacoby R, Levy R. Psychiatric phenomena in Alzheimer's disease. IV: Disorders of behavior. Br J Psychiatry 1990; 157:86–94.

Carlson DL, Fleming KC, Smith GE, Evans JM. Management of dementia-related behavioral disturbances: a non-pharmacologic approach. [Review] Mayo Clin Proc 1995; 70(11):1108–1115.

Devanand DP, Jacobs DM, Tang MX, Del Castillo-Castaneda C, Sano M, Marder K, Bell K, Bylsma FW, Brandt J, Albert M, Stern Y. The course of psychopathologic features in mild to moderate Alzheimer disease. Arch Gen Psychiatry 1997 54:257–263.

Haddad PM, Benbow SM. Sexual problems associated with dementia: part 1: problems and their consequences. Int J Geriatr Psychiatry 1993; 8:547–551.

Lyketsos CG, Corazzini K, Steele C. Mania in Alzheimer's Disease. J Neuropsychiatry Clin Neurosci 1995; 7:350–352.

Marin RS, Fogel BS, Hawkins J, Duffy J, Krupp B. Apathy: a treatable syndrome. J Neuropsychiatry Clin Neurosci 1995; 7(1):23–30.

Patel V, Hope T. Aggressive behavior in elderly people with dementia: a review. Int J Geriatr Psychiatry 1993; 8:457–472.

Price TR, McAllister TW. Safety and efficacy of ECT in depressed patients with dementia: a review of clinical experience. Convulsive Ther 1989; 5:1–74.

Rao V, Lyketsos CG. Delusions in Alzheimer's disease. J Neuropsychiatry Clin Neurosci 1998; 10:373–382.

Rovner BW, Steele CD, Shmuely Y, Folstein MF. A randomized trial of dementia care in nursing homes. J Am Geriatr Soc 1996: 44(1):7–13.

Teri L, Wagner A. Alzheimer's disease and depression. J Consult Clin Psychol 1992; 60:379–391.

Wagner AW, Terri L, Orr-Rainey N. Behavior problems of residents with dementia in special care units. Alzheimer Dis Assoc Disord 1995; 9:121–127.

CHAPTER 9: NONCOGNITIVE BEHAVIORAL AND PSYCHIATRIC DISORDERS

Fitten LJ, Perryman K, Wilkinson C, Little RJ, Burns MM, Pachana N, Mervis JR, Malmgren R, Siembieda, DW, Ganzell S. Alzheimer and vascular dementias and driving. JAMA 1995; 273:1360–1365.

Hall GR. Chronic dementia: challenges in feeding a patient. J Gerontol Nurs 1994; 20:21–30.

Robinson A, Spencer B, White L. Understanding difficult behaviors. Geriatric Education Center of Michigan, Michigan Department of Mental Hygiene, 1988.

Sloane PD, Rader J, Barrick AL, Hoeffer B, Dwyere S, McKenzie D, Lavelle M, Buckwalter K, Arrington L, Pruitt T. Bathing persons with dementia. Gerontologist 1995; 35:672–678.

CHAPTER 10: PHARMACOLOGIC AND OTHER BIOLOGIC TREATMENTS IN DEMENTIA

Burgio LD, Reynolds CF, Janoski JE. A behavioral microanalysis of the effects of haloperidol and oxazepam in demented psychogeriatric inpatients. Int J Geriatr Psychiatry 1992; 7:253–262.

Carlyle W, Ancill RJ, Sheldon L. Aggression in the demented patient: a double-blind study of loxapine versus haloperidol. Int Clin Psychopharmacol 1993; 8:103–108.

Cummings JL, Gorman DG, Shapira J. Physostigmine ameliorates the delusions of Alzheimer's disease. Biol Psychiatry 1993; 33:536–541.

Gottlieb GL, McAllister TW, Gus RC. Depot neuroleptic in the treatment of behavioral disorders in patients with Alzheimer's disease. J Am Geriatr Soc 1988; 36:642–644.

Kawas C, Resnick S, Morrison A, Brookmeyer R, Corrada M, Zonderman A, Bacal C, Donnell Lingle D, Metter E. A prospective study of estrogen replacement therapy and the risk of developing Alzheimer's disease: The Baltimore Longitudinal Study of Aging. Am Acad Neurol 1997; 48:1517–1521.

Kyomen HH, Mobel KW, Wei JY. The use of estrogen to decrease aggressive physical behavior in elderly men with dementia. J Am Geriatr Soc 1991; 39:1110–1112.

Mellow AM, Solano-Lopez C, Davis S. Sodium valproate in the treatment of behavioral disturbance in dementia. J Geriatr Psychiatry Neurol 1993; 6:205–209.

Mishima K, Okawa M, Kishikawa Y, Hozumi S, Hori H, Takahashi K. Morning bright light therapy for sleep and behavior disorders in elderly patients with dementia. Acta Psychiatr Scand 1994; 89:1–7.

Nyth AL, Gottfries CG. The clinical efficacy of citalopram in treatment of emotional disturbances of dementia subjects. Br J Psychiatry 1990; 157:894–901.

Ott BR. Leuprolide treatment of sexual aggression in a patient with dementia and the Kluver-Bucy syndrome. Clin Neuropharmacol 1995; 18:443–447.

Petracca G, Teson A, Chemerinski E, Leiguarda R, Startstein SE. A double-blind placebo controlled study of chlomipramine in depressed patients with Alzheimer's disease. J Neuropsychiatry Clin Neurosci 1996; 8:27–275.

Reifler BV, Teri L, Raskind M, Veith R, Barnes R, White E, McLean P. Double blind trial of imipramine in Alzheimer's disease patients with and without depression. Am J Psychiatry 1989; 146:45–49.

Steele C, Lucas M, Tune L. Haloperidol vs. thioridazine in the treatment of behavioral disturbances in patients with Alzheimer's disease. J Clin Psychiatry 1986; 47:310–312.

Targano FE, Lyketsos CG, Mangone CA, Allegri RF, Comesaña-Diaz E. Double-blind, randomized, fixed dose trial of fluoxetine versus amitriptyline in the treatment of major depression complicating Alzheimer's disease. Psychosomatics 197; 38:246–252.

Tariot PN, Erb R, Liebovici A, Podgorski CA, Cox C, Asnis J, Kolassa J, Irving C.

Carbamazepine treatment of agitation in nursing home patients with dementia: a preliminary study. J Am Geriatr Soc 1994; 42(11): 1160–1166.

CHAPTER 11: TERMINAL CARE

Andrews M, Bell ER, Smith SA, Tischler JF, Veglia JM. Dehydration in terminally ill patients. Postgrad Med 1993; 93:201–208.
Bergstrom N, Braden B, Kemp M, Champagne M, Ruby E. Multi-site study of incidence of pressure ulcers and the relationship between risk level, demographic characteristics, diagnoses, and prescription of preventive interventions. J Am Geriatr Soc 1996; 44:22–30.
Fabiszewski KJ, Volicer B, Volicer L. Effect of antibiotic treatment on outcome of fevers in institutionalized Alzheimer patients. JAMA 1990; 263:3168–3172.
Fabisziewski KJ, Riley ME, Berkley D, Karner J, Shea S. Management of advanced Alzheimer dementia. In Volicer L, Fabisziewski KJ, Rheaume YL, Lash KE, Editors, Clinical Management of Alzheimer's Disease, Aspen: Rockville, 1988.
Hanrahan P, Luchins DJ. Access to hospice programs in end-stage dementia: a national survey of hospice programs. J Am Geriatr Soc 1995; 43:56–59.
Standards and Accreditation Committee-Medical Guidelines Task Force. Medical guidelines for determining prognosis in selected non-cancer diseases. National Hospice Organization: Arlington, VA, 1996.
Stern Y, Tang MX, Albert MS, Brandt J, Jacobs DM, Bell K, Marder K, Sano M, Devanand D, Albert SM, Bylsma F, Tsai WY. Predicting time to nursing home care and death in individuals with Alzheimer's disease. JAMA 1997; 277: 806–813.
Volicer BJ, Hurley A, Fabiszewski KJ, Montgomery P, Volicer L. Predicting short-term survival for patients with advanced Alzheimer's disease. J Am Geriatr Soc 1993; 41:535–540.

CHAPTER 12: ETHICAL AND LEGAL ISSUES

Jonsen A, Siegler M, Winslade WJ. Clinical Ethics. McMillan: New York, 1982.
Norberg A, Hirschfeld M, Davidson B, Davis A, Lauri S, Lin JY, Phillips L, Pittmen E, Vander Laan R, Ziv L. Ethical reasoning concerning the feeding of severely demented patients: an international perspective. Nursing Ethics 1994; 1:3–13.
Post SG. The Moral Challenge of Alzheimer Disease. Johns Hopkins Press: Baltimore, 1995.

CHAPTER 13: CLINICAL GENETICS AND DEMENTIA

Lendon CL, Ashall F, Goate AM. Exploring the etiology of Alzheimer disease using molecular genetics. JAMA 1997; 277:825–831.
Connor JM, Ferguson-Smith MA. Essential Medical Genetics. Blackwell Scientific: London, 1984.
Marx J. New gene tied to common form of Alzheimer's. Science 1988; 281:507–509.

Index

Page references followed by the letter '*f*' refer to figures.
Page references followed by the letter '*t*' refer to tables.